VIRUSES AND PANDEMICS

2020 Edition

Frank Muller

Table of Contents

INTRODUCTION

Coronaviruses (COV) are a Big Family of germs that cause illness, which range from the frequent cold to more serious diseases like Middle East Respiratory Syndrome (MERS-COV) and Severe Acute Respiratory Syndrome (SARS-COV). A novel coronavirus (COV) is a new breed that hasn't been previously recognized in people.

Coronaviruses are zoonotic, which means They're transmitted between people and animals. Thorough investigations discovered that SARS-COV was sent by civet cats to individuals and MERS-COV by dromedary camels to people. Many famous coronaviruses are circulating in creatures that haven't been infected people.

Frequent Indications of the disease include Respiratory symptoms, fever, fever, shortness of breath, and breathing problems. In more serious cases, the infection can lead to pneumonia, severe acute respiratory illness, kidney failure, and even death.

Standard recommendations to stop Disease spread comprise routine hand washing, covering nose and mouth when coughing and coughing, thoroughly cooking eggs and meat. Avoid close contact with anyone displaying symptoms of respiratory disease, including coughing and coughing.

Observing the Initial reports of instances of respiratory syndrome at the Oriental Wuhan municipality at the end of December 2019, Chinese governments have recognized a novel coronavirus as the key causative agent. The epidemic has quickly evolved, influencing different elements of China and away from the nation. Examples have been found in many nations in Asia, but also in Australia, Europe, Africa, and North America. The initial cases from the EU/EEA have been verified in France. The further worldwide spread is anticipated.

About 12 February 2020, the publication Coronavirus was called severe acute respiratory syndrome coronavirus two (SARS-CoV-2), whereas the disorder connected with it has become known as COVID-19. It's a new breed of coronavirus which hasn't been previously recognized in people. Outbreaks of publication virus infections among individuals are constantly of public health issues, particularly when there's minimal understanding about the qualities of the virus and how it propagates between individuals, how intense would be the consequent ailments, and how to deal with them.

The human-to-human transmission was Verified, but more info is required to assess the complete scope of the manner of transmission. The origin of the disease is unknown and may continue to be active.

This can be an Emerging, rapidly evolving scenario with continuing outbreak investigations. ECDC is closely tracking this epidemic and providing risk evaluations to direct the EU Member States and the EU Commission within their response actions.

Regular hazard assessment on COVID-19

The danger related to COVID-19 Disease for men and women in the EU/EEA and the UK is now regarded as moderate.

This evaluation relies on the following variables:

- Most cases reported at the EU/EEA, along with the UK out a few areas in Italy, have recognized epidemiological connections. But, there's a growing amount of instances with no specified series of transmission. Outstanding general health measures are employed in Italy and other EU/EEA and the UK, and solid efforts have been forced to identify, isolate, and examine contacts so as to contain the epidemic. However, in spite of touch tracing measures started to include additional spread, there are still exportations and also an increasing number of sporadic instances across EU/EEA nations. The likelihood of additional transmission at the EU/EEA along with the UK is regarded as moderate to large. There's still a degree of uncertainty concerning many unpredictable things in a situation that's still evolving.

- The chance of new connections from some other nations outside China to the EU/EEA seems to be rising as the number of countries reporting instances keeps moving up. A thorough collection of those countries is available here. This also raises the chance of instances being released by travellers from different countries outside China into the EU/EEA and UK.

- The evidence accumulated thus far in the investigation of COVID-19 instances is that COVID-19 disease causes moderate illness (i.e., non-pneumonia or moderate infections) in roughly 80 percent of cases. More serious disease happens in about 20 percent of cases, together with roughly one in four or even five undergoing significant illness. The excellent majority of the very severe kinds of disease, and fatalities, have occurred among the elderly, especially those with other chronic diseases.

The Danger of the incidence of Clusters, like the people in Italy, correlated with COVID-19 from different nations in the EU/EEA along with the UK is now regarded as moderate to large.

This evaluation relies on the following variables:

- The present event in Italy suggests that local transmission could have resulted in many clusters. They gathered evidence from clusters declared from the EU/EEA, and the UK suggests that after compressed, the virus resulting in COVID-19 could be transmitted quickly. It's plausible that a percentage of transmissions happen from cases with moderate symptoms that don't provoke healthcare-seeking behavior. The increase in case numbers and the Amount of countries beyond China reporting these instances raises the possible avenues of importation of this disease into the EU/EEA along with the United Kingdom. Importations from several other European nations have already happened.

- The effects of these clusters at the EU/EEA are high, particularly if hospitals had been changed, and also a high number of health care employees had to be dispersed. The effect on vulnerable groups from the hospitals or health care facilities is acute, specifically for the older.

- The stringent general public health measures which were implemented immediately following distinguishing the German COVID-19 instances will decrease but not eliminate the likelihood of additional spread.

The Danger of individuals from the EU/EEA As well as the UK traveling/resident in both regions having supposed community transmission is presently large.

This evaluation relies on the following variables:

- The general number of documented instances in most areas with community transmission is either increasing or high. Nevertheless, there are important doubts regarding transmissibility and under-detection, especially among moderate or asymptomatic circumstances.
- For travellers/residents, the evidence accumulated up to now from an investigation of COVID-19 instances is that COVID-19 disease causes moderate illness (i.e., non-pneumonia or moderate ailments) in roughly 80 percent of cases. More serious disease happens in about 20 percent of cases, together with roughly one in four or even five undergoing significant illness. The excellent majority of the very severe kinds of disease, and fatalities, have occurred among the elderly, especially those with other chronic diseases.

The Danger of health care systems Capability from the EU/EEA and also the UK throughout the continuing influenza season is deemed moderate right now.

This evaluation relies on the following variables:

- Since the amount of documented COVID-19 instances from the EU/EEA along with the UK is rising, the likelihood of widespread disease is rising from low to average throughout the continuing 2019--2020 flu season. Nearly all states reported widespread flu activity per week 7/2020; however, the ratio of specimens tested positive in sentinel surveillance is marginally diminishing; a few EU/EEA nations might have moved beyond the summit period of elevated flu circulation. For the most recent flu update, see the combined ECDC--WHO/Europe weekly flu update.

- In case a substantial growth in COVID-19 instances was to coincide with a high amount of flu activity, the possible effect on health care systems could be moderate to large. The greater variety of instances would call for extra funds such as testing, case reporting, surveillance, and contact tracing. Greater transmission could cause additional strain on health care systems. This scenario will be exacerbated if a Significant amount of healthcare workers become infected

There's a spread of a publication Coronavirus that's wreaking havoc around the town of Wuhan situated in the Hubei province of China. The epidemic of this virus started early in December of 2019 and has since continued to propagate. The men and women that had been the primary ones to eventually become infected were linked into this South China Seafood Wholesale Market that has been closed since.

Thousands of instances have been reported by health officials in China. Additionally, there are instances which were identified in different nations, largely spread from the folks traveling from China, such as Chinese individuals or the folks returning from China for their own various nations. The virus may spread from 1 individual to another via contact or perhaps simply being in the proximity of the infected individual.

More than 20 nations have reported Cases, such as Singapore, Japan, Hong Kong, Thailand, Malaysia, South Korea, Taiwan, Germany, Vietnam, Australia, France, the USA, India, the united kingdom, etc., and a number of different nations have put up screening facilities for those coming from China.

That can be a big family of viruses That are jointly called the coronavirus. The majority of the recognized coronavirus symptoms just have easy impacts on the people like providing them a moderate respiratory disease such as the frequent cold; however, there are two such instances of this coronavirus which have shown enormous results on the infected that can be Severe Acute Respiratory Syndrome (SARS) coronavirus and also Middle East Respiratory Syndrome (MERS) coronavirus.

Symptoms:

Fever, coughing, and problem Breathing are a number of the symptoms and signs that have been found from the individuals infected. A few of the patients also have reported with a sore throat. There has been some speculation concerning the acute disease-causing possibility of this novel coronavirus though these claims aren't supported with appropriate proof. Individuals with chronic diseases and elderly patients may pose higher odds of giving birth to severe illness as a consequence of this virus.

Risk

The Men and Women That Are alive or Traveling across the region where the virus is more widespread are at a higher risk of disease based on the WHO. Presently, the virus is just within China, and each one of the non-residents of China who've been infected travelled to China lately and has already related to the contaminated men and women that are out of China.

Thus, in accordance with WHO, the threat to the men and women that aren't residing in China is quite low provided that you do not come in contact with a few of those non-resident Chinese men and women that are infected. Additionally, the WHO claims that easy disinfectants can quickly eliminate this virus if it's found on a surface as well as the survival period of this virus onto any surface is really low.

Conclusion:

This informative article discusses all the Symptoms to consider if you believe you may be impacted by the virus; however, if you are a non-resident and have been connected with anybody traveling from China, then you don't have any possibility of catching the virus."

A Deadly Contagious Airborne Disease (Coronavirus)

Coronavirus, also Called SARS-COV, Was accountable to the deadly SARS (Severe Acute Respiratory Syndrome) outbreak in Asia in 2003 along with the virus immediately went across boundaries and caused secondary situations, triggering a global state of fear with the epidemic of this illness turned right into a worldwide epidemic. SARS is a fatal and infectious airborne disease. Passing can be as quick as in 24 hours from contaminated men and women.

Tired of authorities scrambled to Hold meetings, along with the authorities of China (where the epidemic allegedly started) took quite aggressive steps to suppress and contain the illness, such as shutting down businesses, schools, and offices, and enforced a 30 days house rewired because of the taxpayers. The efforts paid off, and also on 18 May 2004, the epidemic was announced to have been contained.

The World Health Organization (WHO) Recommends immediate isolation for many suspected and likely instances of SARS in an attempt to curtail the spread since it minimizes contact with different men and women.

But, for caretakers of the ill Patients with flu-like indicators of suspected SARS cases, a few homecare preventative measures have to be taken, so the entire family residing in precisely the exact same home isn't infected also.

The individual could be given a different room from the remainder of the household, to recover. Home and personal hygiene have to be turned up with cleaning activities like washing machines, washing clothing, and cleansing the ground to keep the surroundings clean. If at all possible, install a fantastic air purifier that could ruin and reduce the quantity of coronavirus flying around in the atmosphere, which may infect another household member.

CHAPTER ONE
THE HISTORY OF CORONAVIRUS

Coronaviruses are a group of viruses that cause disorders in birds and mammals. In people, coronaviruses cause respiratory tract ailments, which are generally moderate, like the frequent cold, although milder forms like SARS, MERS, and also COVID-19 could be deadly. Symptoms change in different species: chickens, they create an upper respiratory tract infection, while in cattle and pigs, they trigger diarrhea. There are to be vaccines or antiviral medications to prevent or cure human coronavirus infections.

Coronaviruses include the subfamily Orthocoronavirinae from the family Coronaviridae, at the order Nidovirales. They have enveloped viruses with a positive-sense single-stranded RNA genome and a nucleocapsid of helical symmetry. The genome size of coronaviruses ranges from roughly 27 to 34 kilobases, the biggest one of the famous RNA viruses. The title coronavirus comes from the Latin corona, meaning "crown" or "halo," which relates to the characteristic look of these virus particles (virions): they got a fringe reminiscent of a crown or of a solar corona.

Coronaviruses were found in the 1960s. The first ones found have been infectious bronchitis virus from chickens and 2 viruses in the sinus cavities of individual patients with the frequent cold, which were then called human coronavirus 229E and human coronavirus OC43. [9] Additional members of the family have been recognized, such as SARS-COV at 2003, HCOV NL63 in 2004, respectively HKU1 at 2005," MERS-COV at 2012, along with SARS-CoV-2 (previously called 2019-nCoV) in 2019; many of them have been included in acute respiratory tract ailments.

Title and morphology

The title "coronavirus" will be Derived in the Latin corona as well as also the Greek κορώνη (korónē,"garland, wreath"), significance crown or halo. The title describes the characteristic look of virions (the infective form of the virus) by electron microscopy that includes a fringe of big, bulbous surface projections producing a picture reminiscent of a crown or using a solar corona. This morphology is made by the viral spike (S) peplomers, which are proteins on the surface of the virus, which decide host tropism.

Proteins that Lead to the general construction of coronaviruses are the spike (S), envelope (E), membrane (M), and nucleocapsid (N). In the particular instance of the SARS coronavirus (see under), a specified receptor-binding domain name on S mediates the attachment of the virus into the cell receptor, angiotensin-converting receptor 2 (ACE2). Some coronaviruses (especially the associates of Beta coronavirus subgroup A) have a briefer spike-like protein called hemagglutinin esterase (HE).

Replication

After entry to the host cell, the Virus particle is uncoated, and its own genome enters the cell cytoplasm.

The coronavirus RNA genome includes a 5′ Methylated cap plus a 3′ polyadenylated tail, allowing the RNA to attach into the host cell's ribosome for translation.

Coronavirus genomes also simplify a Protein known as RNA-dependent RNA polymerase (RDRP), which permits the viral genome to be invisible to fresh RNA copies utilizing the host cell's machines. The RDRP is the first protein to be produced; after that, the gene encoding the RDRP is interpreted; translation has been stopped by a stop codon. This is referred to as a nested transcript. After the mRNA transcript only encodes one particular gene, it's monoisotopic. Coronavirus non-structural proteins deliver additional fidelity into replication since they exude a function, which can be lacking RNA-dependent RNA polymerase enzymes independently.

The genome is duplicated along with a long Polyprotein is shaped, in which all the proteins have been attached. Coronaviruses have a non-structural protein, a protease -- that can cleave the polyprotein. This procedure is a sort of hereditary market, permitting the virus to synthesize the best number of enzymes in a few nucleotides.

Transmission

Human to human transmission of Coronaviruses is mainly considered to happen among close connections through respiratory droplets made by coughing and coughing.

The Background

Ahead of the novel coronavirus Outbreak struck Wuhan in December, the precise whereabouts -- as well as presence -- of the Chinese town had slid from the public's consciousness from the West.

Nevertheless, it was not always the way.

Two generations ago, this town of 11 Million individuals, at the intersection of the Yangtze and Han Rivers, 600 miles upstream, in central China, has been understood throughout the West as a significant industrial town.

It was someplace many European Forces needed a consulate, a location where leading Japanese and Western trading companies, and global textile and technology businesses, had factories and sales offices.

It was a frequent overseas posting for customs officials, steamboat captains, dealers, and consuls. Wuhan was a cradle of China's revolution in 1911. A quarter of a century later, it stood as the beleaguered wartime funding of governmental China.

In the Centre of the 19th century Before the center of the 20th century, the Wuhan turned into a town which frequently appeared in the global media and, as a trading hub for both teas and silks one of the other commodities, it immediately influenced the lives of men and women in the West -- it created the tea into their teapots the roasted egg within their own birthday cakes the silk to get their own pajamas.

Following the destruction and chaos of That the Second World War, the Communist Revolution introduced the Bamboo Curtain ardently down. Worldwide trade ceased, the foreign exchange community abandoned, along with the Western world, mostly whined about Wuhan.

The Chicago of all China

Back in 1900, American magazine Collier's Published a post concerning the Yangtze "boom town" of Wuhan, calling it "the Chicago of China." It had been among those very first instances -- maybe not the very first -- that the Chinese town was awarded that this moniker, and it stuck.

Back in 1927, the veteran United Press Shanghai correspondent Randall Gould used the moniker at a shipment about political chaos in Hubei province. Next, the expression appears countless times in only about every single paper round world.

Minnesota-born Gould was rather Fresh off the ship in Shanghai once he awakened the Yangtze to Wuhan for the very first time. Gould was in the city since a revolution was happening -- that the next in Wuhan within 15 decades. Meanwhile, the Nationalist government, headed by Chiang Kai-shek, had divided within the damn suppression tactics utilized in its own brutal war against the Communist Party.

A steamer is packed with Hankow.

Left-wing sympathizers based The Wuhan Nationalist Government, although Chiang formed his own bulk government in Nanjing. The alternate authorities in Wuhan just lasted six weeks, but it showed that the long-running branches within the Nationalist Party. To overseas correspondents such as Gould, it seemed just like the youthful Chinese republic was going to wrench itself aside.

Their editors from London, New York, Paris, and Tokyo agreed. Wuhan was the news.

That editorial conclusion was partially Affected by the very long list of firms with large bets in Wuhan in 1927 -- both the Hong Kong & Shanghai Bank (HSBC), John Swire & Sons, British-American Tobacco, Standard Oil of New York, Texaco, Standard Chartered Bank.

Wuhan has been China's leading industrial Powerhouse, making steel and iron, cotton and silk, tea packaging, and food canning.

This was the Chicago of all China.

The West's debut to Wuhan

The West came to understand Wuhan in 1858 As a portion of this unequal Treaty of Tianjin, expressed by the reduced Qing Dynasty through the Second Opium War.

The treaty permitted foreign boats to Sail the Yangtze River, and also, the British had researched the waterway so far as Hubei province. They especially studied the riverside conglomeration of Wuchang, Hankou, and Hanyang jointly called the "Three Towns of Wuhan." Liking what they watched, they needed that the town is exposed to foreign exchange.

Robert Bickers, a professor in Bristol University, who research the international exchange in pre-1949 China, describes that the British believing: "Following the First Opium War that the British annexed Hong Kong as a colony and also opened Shanghai, on the shore at the heart of the Yangtze in southern China, as a treaty port. Sixteen decades after they knew the significance of inland China improved and zeroed on Wuhan, in addition to Tianjin."

Wuhan became crucial to this Coastal port towns, feeding them products (tea, beef, java, etc.) and Produced outputs (steel, iron, silk). Wuhan has been China's biggest inland entrepôt.

Wuhan Was a gigantic in town in 1850 -- roughly 1 million individuals lived in the 3 cities half of the magnitude of the world's biggest city at that moment, London.

In the 1860s, Thieves Bombarded In, although the city constantly had a Chinese bulk inhabitant.

The new arrivals indulged in Hankou Developing a coastal, two-mile extended Bund that mostly remains now, constructing their houses, docks, and workplaces in addition to a race track, clubs, and general gardens all adjoining to the Hankou shore.

The British Concession was adjoining to concessions run from the Germans, the French, the Japanese, also a somewhat contested Belgian concession, along with the Russians, that was busy in Wuhan trading prohibited out of Siberia as the 12th century. These states, such as the Americans, had consulates. Holt House has been the workplace to Butterfield & Swire, among the most significant and most bizarre British"hongs" or trading homes in China.

Even though Wuhan turned into a cosmopolitan Location, it was almost always fundamentally a company city -- it had acquired the nightlife or even the film business, publishing houses, and art galleries which surfaced in Shanghai's more Bohemian quarters; it was not rather the scholarly center that has been Beijing. The thieves were current, and also their soldiers defeated the consulates; however, the town kept a much dominant Chinese sense.

Facility of revolt

Back in 1911, the republican revolution That overthrew China's last imperial dynasty has been accidental, sparked in Wuhan.

The first catalyst for its revolt Was the accidental explosion of a bomb that happened when a careless anti-Qing/pro-republican radical dropped a lit cigarette at the workshop of rebel conspirators at Hankou's Russian Concession.

The consequent explosion alerted a Nervous German butcher who telephoned the authorities, who subsequently discovered a plot that was revolutionary. Seals, programs, and papers were captured implicating members of their town's Wuchang Garrison of Chinese soldiers since revolutionaries preparing to mutiny. As authorities had captured their membership record, the rebels were confronted with a decision between torture, arrest, and likely beheading or setting up a struggle. They made a decision to act quickly to maintain themselves.

The anti-Qing rebellion took the record and finished the 267-year-old Qing Dynasty.

Generally, foreign Enterprise Welcomed the new republic and watched it as a harbinger of higher service for modern businesses.

Really, Wuhan was awash with fresh Industrial suggestions and technology. The town was home to many leading Chinese heavy businesses -- that the Hubei Arsenal and Powder functions, Hanyang Iron and Steel, a railroad to Beijing, routine steamer solutions to Shanghai, a bulk of silk filatures, cotton mills and canneries. The town's furnaces created a large proportion of the planet's horseshoes -- an item as crucial from the late 19th century since tires now.

Its inventory yards boiled pig down Carcasses from the countless thousands to extract countless pig bristles for export to Europe and America -- both the important and crucial, element from the thriving toothbrush marketplace. Wuhan was also a middle of egg production -- new eggs, maintained, roasted, liquid -- also exported them into food producers, restaurants, and bakeries across the planet.

Since Wuhan became industrially Significant internationally, its position as an export power gave the town federal electricity.

Robert Bickers notes the town "unobtrusively entered customers' lives in Europe and America." However, some overseas buyers did not feel that China could create steel, iron, and meals to Western criteria.

Nevertheless, China was fabricating steel and iron to get its railways, bridges, and urban structure whilst at the same time ramping up its armaments sector to make a newly-organized contemporary military beneath Chiang Kai-shek's command. Ways about these overseas prejudices needed to be discovered. Comparatively low prices were just one approach to convince low-income buyers others had been a bit more imaginative.

CHAPTER TWO
OVERVIEW OF CORONAVIRUS

Coronaviruses cause a significant Percent of human deaths and a slew of frequent respiratory ailments in a number of different creatures, such as economically significant diseases of poultry, livestock, and lab rodents. Additionally, though these viruses weren't known for generating over moderate infections in humans before the SARS outbreak, furry coronavirologists have been conscious of the possibility of generating deadly ailments in animals, even as Linda Saif clarifies in this chapter's original newspaper. Because of this, there's an extensive quantity of research on animal coronaviruses which could be drawn out for understanding the life cycle and pathogenicity of the SARS virus, and also veterinary scientists ' are presently being called to join the study response to the outbreak and discuss their understanding of coronaviruses using a wider audience. Mark Denison's newspaper describes the present state of research on animal coronaviruses and discusses results from these types of animal models indicate promising directions for future study about SARS and other emerging zoonoses.

Animal coronaviruses are inclined to follow Among two fundamental pathogenic versions, making enteric or respiratory ailments. Both models reveal parallels to the ecological characteristics of SARS patients, the vast majority of those presented with respiratory ailments, but in a few instances also endured from thyroid complications. In mature animals, coronavirus diseases of a respiratory character have revealed improved severity in the existence of many aspects, such as elevated exposure levels, respiratory coinfections, anxiety linked to transport or commingling with creatures from other farms, and therapy with corticosteroids. In youthful, seronegative creatures, enteric coronaviruses may lead to deadly infections. Though coronaviruses normally result in illness in one animal species, a few have now been proven to cross species barriers.

Substantial effort has been Applied toward discovering an animal origin of the SARS virus. This was sought mainly throughout the genetic characterization of viral isolates from supposed animal resources compared to individual SARS coronavirus samples. In years past nevertheless, epidemiological detective work has recognized the origin of several outbreaks of infectious illness, and yet another workshop participant indicated a case-control analysis of the initial 50 to 100 SARS patients in China's Guangdong Province, in which the oldest cases of this disease have been discovered, could prove similarly successful. Even though a natural reservoir for the SARS virus hasn't yet been recognized, the blend of these genomic and epidemiological methods is already affording suggestive outcomes. By way of instance, the previous paper in this chapter by Yi Guan et al. clarifies the existence of coronaviruses closely associated with

SARS, one of the live animals offered in Guangdong markets. Similar epidemiological principles could nevertheless offer valuable direction for additional lab polls of animal viruses geared toward discovering the initial reservoir and source of the SARS coronavirus.

Coronaviruses have been categorized into three main categories according to their genetic traits. Though the SARS virus was connected with Group II coronaviruses, whose associates consist of human and bovine respiratory ailments as well as also the mouse hepatitis virus, there's still some disagreement over if its genetic attributes may be sufficiently different to justify classification within another, the fourth category of coronaviruses. Studies of coronavirus replication at the molecular level show several mechanisms that account for the recurrent, persistent infections average of coronaviral disease. High levels of mutation and also RNA-RNA recombination create viruses that can adapt to obtain and recover virulence. Even though researchers have identified many possible targets for antifungal treatments, the capability of the virus to mutate and recombine signifies a significant barrier to embryo development. A vaccine that may provide highly powerful, long-term defense from respiratory coronavirus infections hasn't been developed, nor possess proper animal continues to be designed to examine potential vaccines against SARS. It was mentioned by many workshop participants a coordinated, multidisciplinary study campaign, drawing on experience in the biomedical and veterinary sciences, will probably be required to fulfil these aims.

Coronaviruses are a big family of Viruses, a few of which cause sickness in humans, and many others which circulate among birds and mammals. Paradoxically, animal coronaviruses may spread to people, then spread between individuals. Zoonotic coronaviruses have emerged in the last several years to induce human outbreaks like COVID-19, severe acute respiratory syndrome (SARS), and also Middle East respiratory disease (MERS).

Infection in humans mostly manifests as respiratory disease, or occasionally gastrointestinal disease. The clinical spectrum of disease changes from no symptoms or mild respiratory ailments to acute, rapidly progressive illness, severe respiratory distress syndrome, septic shock, or multi-organ collapse is leading to death.

What's a coronavirus, and what should I do if I have symptoms?

What's Covid-19 -- the disease which Began in Wuhan?

It's Brought on by a member of this Coronavirus family that has never been struck before. Like other coronaviruses, it has come out of creatures. Many of the originally infected either worked or regularly shopped from the Huanan fish wholesale marketplace in the middle of the Chinese town.

Which are the symptoms this coronavirus causes?

The virus may lead to pneumonia. Those Who have fallen sick are reported to endure coughs, fever, and breathing problems. In acute cases, there may be organ collapse. As this can be a viral disease, antibiotics are of no use. The antiviral medications we have against influenza won't get the job done. Recovery is based upon the potency of their immune system. A lot of those people who have perished were in bad health.

If I go to the doctor whenever I have A cough?

In the United Kingdom, the medical information is That if you've recently travelled from regions impacted by a coronavirus, you need to:

- remain inside and avoid contact with different people as you want the influenza
- telephone NHS 111 to notify them of your latest travel into the region

How many individuals are affected?

On 1 March, the epidemic has Influenced an estimated 87,000 people worldwide. In southern China, there were 2,870 deaths among over 79,000 instances, largely from the central province of Hubei. Over 41,000 individuals affected in China have recovered.

Even the coronavirus has spread at least 30 different nations. The badly affected include Japan, together with 850 instances, such as 691 in the cruise ship docked in Yokohama, along with four deaths. Italy has listed at least 1,100 cases and 29 deaths, whereas South Korea has listed over 3,500 cases and eight deaths. There also have been deaths from Hong Kong, Taiwan, France, the US, and the Philippines.

There were 15 recorded instances and no deaths thus far in the United Kingdom.

Why is this worse than ordinary flu, and how concerned are the specialists?

We do not yet understand how harmful the Brand-new coronavirus, and also we will not know until more information comes from. The mortality rate is about 2% at the epicenter of the epidemic, Hubei state, and much less than this elsewhere. For contrast, seasonal influenza typically includes a mortality rate under 1 percent and is considered to cause roughly 400,000 deaths annually worldwide. SARS had a passing rate of over 10 percent.

Another crucial unknown is the way that Infectious the coronavirus is. An essential distinction is that unlike influenza, there's not any vaccine for its new coronavirus, meaning it's more challenging for vulnerable individuals of their populace -- older people or people with existing respiratory or immune disorders -- to shield themselves. Hand-washing and preventing different people if you're feeling unwell are significant. 1 sensible thing is to have the influenza vaccine, that will cut the load on health services in the event the outbreak turns out to a wider outbreak.

Are there other coronaviruses?

Severe acute respiratory syndrome (SARS) and Middle Eastern respiratory syndrome (MERS) are caused by coronaviruses that originated from creatures. Back in 2002, SARS spread nearly impervious to 37 nations, inducing international terror, infecting more than 8,000 people and killing over 750. MERS seems to be easily passed from human to human, but contains higher lethality, killing 35 percent of roughly 2,500 those who've been infected.

Is the epidemic that a pandemic, and Should we fear?

No. A pandemic, in WHO conditions, is "the global spread of illness." The spread of this virus outside China is stressful but not a sudden improvement. The WHO has announced the outbreak for a public health emergency of global concern. The crucial issues are the way transmissible this new coronavirus is involving individuals, and what percentage become seriously ill and wind up in the hospital. Often viruses that spread readily generally get a milder effect. Normally, the coronavirus seems to be hitting against elderly people toughest, with few instances in children.

Coronavirus outbreak

A SARS-like virus epidemic Located in Wuhan, China, is dispersing neighboring Asian nations, as far afield as Australia, the US, and Europe. What's China and the entire world reacting to this coronavirus outbreak?

Global Data's Most Up-to-date Coronavirus Influencers dash has become live on Pharmaceutical Technology; also it allows you to monitor the most recent developments linked to the coronavirus outbreak and also follow down the activity of major influencers on the outbreak.

29 Feb:

Death toll nears 3,000 globally, and recoveries cross 42,000

-- How many deaths because of Covid-19 is over 2,970, at the end of 29 February.

-- The Complete number of cases raised to over 86,500, with much more 79,824 cases supported at Mainland China. The recoveries also have climbed to over 42,000 worldwide.

-- Mainland China reported 573 brand new cases and 35 deaths.

Iran reports nine brand new deaths

Iran has reported two deaths and 205 confirmed instances, carrying the death toll on 43 and verified instances to 593.

Top of Form

How convinced are you that international Health governments can comprise the Wuhan coronavirus epidemic?

• Unbelievably Optimistic

• Fairly optimistic

• Not convinced

Bottom of Form

South Korea accounts for 376 instances

-- KCDC reports added 376 instances, Taking the amount to 3,526 while the death toll stands at 17.

Australia and Thailand report Deaths

-- A 78-year-old repatriated guy from That the Diamond Princess cruise boat has expired in Australia, the nation's first death instance. The overall cases in the nation remain at 27, such as 2 new confirmed cases.

-- Thailand reported additionally reported Its very first circumstance, reported that the Ministry of Public health. The dead person was a 35-year-old guy who suffered from dengue fever prior to testing positive for coronavirus. The overall cases in Thailand stand in 42.

28 Feb:

The US reports the death

-- The US reported its first departure; The dead person was in his 50s and has been out of Seattle, Washington. He had been reported to have underlying health issues.

-- The US has also improved its Traveling restrictions South Korea, Iran, and Italy because of the rising number of instances in the nations.

First instances documented in Monaco, Mexico along with Azerbaijan

-- A guy from Monaco has already reported that the First instance of Covid-19. The guy is admitted to a hospital in France.

-- Mexico reported its initial two Cases in the nation, one that tested positive and yet another who's expecting test results. The next instance is regarded as verified.

-- Azerbaijan has already reported its original the event of Covid-19. The individual had been from Russia, who came from Iran.

Romania, Denmark, Norway and also Georgia Report new instances

-- Romania has already reported two Additional situations, bringing the total to 3.

-- Denmark affirmed its second Coronavirus instance, a guy who returned in northern Italy.

-- Others have tested positive In Norway, carrying the nation's total cases into four.

-- Georgia has also listed its Second instance of this virus. The girl a 31-years-old and went to Italy.

Singapore affirms four instances of coronavirus

-- Singapore has recently reported Additional situations, taking the total to 102. Singapore's Ministry of Health has included it additionally introduced three instances.

-- The Entire recovered instances from the Nation stands in 72.

South Korea reports added Instances; one passing

-- KCDC has declared 219 additional Instances and one new passing. The nation's death toll stands at 17, while the overall instances are 3,150.

-- Total instances in Iraq have improved to eight while instances in Lebanon endure.

-- A guy who arrived in Israel from Italy has tested positive for Covid-19, bringing the total to seven in the nation.

-- Finland has reported that the Nation's total now stands in three confirmed cases.

-- Bahrain supported two cases of Coronavirus, which is out of Saudi Arabia. The complete in Bahrain stands in 38.

Death toll rises to over 2,900

-- The death toll because of has Increased to over 2,900, at the end of 28 February.

-- The number of verified cases Across the globe has risen to over 85,000, while recoveries stand in 39,000.

South Korea reports added Instances; three deaths

-- South Korea reported yet another 594 Cases, raising the overall cases to 2,931. The death toll reached 16.

Singapore accounts two extra Instances

The Entire number of instances in Singapore has risen to 98, such as both new cases reported now.

About 31 December 2019, the Chinese Police reported that a case of pneumonia with an unidentified origin from Wuhan, Hubei province, into the World Health Organisation (WHO)'s China Office. As an increasing number of cases surfaced, totalling 44 by January, the nation's National Health Commission isolated the virus resulting in congestion and flu-like symptoms and recognized this as a novel coronavirus known to the WHO since 2019-nCoV.

What's coronavirus?

Coronaviruses are a group of viruses That trigger respiratory tract infections, including the frequent cold, but could occasionally be serious, especially for babies, the elderly, and individuals with either weak or compromised immune systems, according to the US Centres for Disease Control and Prevention (CDC).

This viral pathogen was accountable for its Middle East Respiratory Syndrome (MERS) and Severe Acute Respiratory (SARS) outbreaks.

The 2003 SARS outbreak appeared Out of China and has been thought to be accountable for 8,000 instances and about 800 deaths. There has been some controversy regarding the Chinese government's direction and alleged cover from the consequences of this virus.

The first recognized case of MERS Happened in 2012 from Saudi Arabia, and the epidemic was mostly inside the Arabian Peninsula. But there has been a bigger outbreak in the Republic of Korea in 2015, conducted by somebody who'd seen Saudi Arabia, the UAE, and Bahrain. There were roughly 186 cases and 36 deaths from this epidemic.

Which will be the coronavirus symptoms?

Regrettably, the Indicators of 2019-nCoV are much like regular influenza symptoms -- such as fever, and cough, and shortness of breath, making them hard to see. The CDC noted symptoms could emerge between 2- and 14-days following exposure to the virus.

Patients are advised to show Themselves into a health care professional when they have these indicators. For individuals beyond China, they're counselled to do this should they've lately returned in China or have already been connected with somebody else that has exhibited these signs.

After an appointment, the Patient will subsequently undergo laboratory-based diagnostic testing for the virus.

Present Worldwide spread of this virus

According to WHO data, as of 20 January, there have been 282 verified cases of this virus, even 278 of that originated in China, centered around the town of Wuhan and the neighboring area with 258 instances. Of the 278 Chinese scenarios, 51 individuals were seriously sick, 12 were at a vital state, and six deaths were reported by Wuhan.

On 13th January, Thailand reported the very first imported case of 2019-nCoV from somebody who'd belonged to Wuhan. In a week, there has been yet another confirmed case in Thailand and a single instance in Japan and one from the Republic of Korea.

You will find reports of additional Instances in Taiwan and in Australia on 21 January. On 22 January, the US CDC reported that the first instance of 2019-nCoV in the united states, causing the standard S&P 500 indicator to slip 0.3% over the stock exchange, according to the Financial Times.

Between 22 and 29 January, the Disorder continued to spread through Asia -- fresh cases arose in Singapore, Hong Kong, Sri Lanka, Cambodia, Nepal, and Malaysia. The exterior of East Asia, fresh instances have emerged in France, Germany, the UAE, and Canada. Keep up-to-date together with the states changed here.

The UK is to report a situation of 2019-nCoV and is trying to display everybody who has come from Wuhan because of mid-January.

The Chinese government estimated that on 22 January, there have been too many as 453 instances on the mainland and also three additional deaths in Hubei province, bringing the complete death toll to eight. As of 29 January, the amount of cases worldwide has reached 6,000, and also the amount of deaths has surpassed 100.

What's the coronavirus delivered?

Although originally it was believed This 2019-nCoV was distributed only through contact with animals since the origin of the epidemic was thought to be a fish and live animal market in Wuhan, Chinese police have confirmed the coronavirus may also be spread via human-to-human contact.

Germany and Japan have verified Domestic transmission of this virus by someone who had lately visited Wuhan to a person who hadn't seen town or China generally.

Reacting to the coronavirus Outbreak

Because of the quick spread of the disease from folks traveling by Wuhan, the town's government has imposed travel restrictions on individuals with congestion or symptoms that are adverse.

The Chinese national government has Implemented similar journey warnings and limitations in the series up to the Lunar New Year parties during the weekend of 25 and 26 January. Infrared thermometers are installed in airports, railroad stations, long-distance travel stations, and ferry terminals.

In an overview about the China National Health Commission's site, Chinese President Xi Jinping stated "all-purpose attempts have to be produced in the prevention and management of their contagion," also called "party committees and governments at different levels in addition to relevant departments to create people's lifestyles and health a priority, devise meticulous programs, mobilize all available sources and also take concrete and effective steps to contain the additional spread of this illness."

The Chinese government also shared that the Genetic arrangement of 2019-nCoV early in January to encourage the identification of possible patients across the planet, in addition to helping the invention of vaccines from this publication virus.

Global Data infectious diseases Analyst Philipp Rosenbaum composed in a business Comment Wire: "Quick identification of germs and data sharing are critical to permit international surveillance to include the spread of this disease, particularly during the continuing cold and flu season, because coronavirus infections originally reveal similar symptoms for respiratory-related hospitalizations because of influenza and cold."

Additionally, the government in the Central province of Henan, which supposes the Hubei state where the epidemic started have prohibited the sale of fish in an effort to stop animal-to-human disperse of 2019-nCoV.

Other Nations Also Have started Screening passengers coming from China and Hong Kong to get 2019-nCoV -- that the US started screening during its key hub airports around 21 January. Additionally, the Financial Times has reported that Russia has fortified controls around its over 4,000km border with China.

WHO's reaction to this outbreak

On 22 January, the WHO convened a Crisis assembly, which the Chinese government will attend to talk about if the 2019-nCoV epidemic ought to be hailed as a public health crisis and what guidelines should be created in the best way best to handle the status.

The WHO chose not to yet announce This outbreak an international health care crisis; however, the supranational body has significantly improved its evaluation of the worldwide threat from medium to high.

The organization's senior leadership team, headed by director-general Dr. Tedros Adhanom Ghebreyesus, held a meeting with Chinese President Xi Jinping on 28 January. The 2 parties shared up-to-date info concerning the condition of the outbreak and also the way they could work together to boost containment -- that the WHO consented to ship global specialists into China to encourage additional evaluations of the harshness of the continuing outbreak and supply advice on continuing avoidance and management efforts.

The WHO also has lasted Communicating with and counselling other nations that are dealing with examples of coronavirus. Furthermore, it has established the worldwide 2019-nCoV Clinical Information Platform to notify global public health reactions to this outbreak.

Vaccines and drugs in the gut for 2019-nCoV

Presently, there's a focus on Avoidance and controlling the spread of the novel coronavirus since there aren't any particular therapy possibilities offered for this specific strain of this virus.

But, lots of researchers and Organizations are employing the genetic code of virus introduced with the Chinese authorities to encourage the growth of vaccines, especially against 2019-nCoV.

The Norway-based Coalition for Epidemic Preparedness Innovations (CEPI) is 1 set leading the area. It's financed three jobs -- one by Inovio, the next with all the Australian University of Queensland and the third party using Moderna, that will work together with the US National Institutes of Health and National Institutes of Allergy and Infectious diseases.

CEPI CEO Richard Hatchett remarked: "Given that the rapid international spread of this nCoV-2019 virus that the entire world should act fast and in readiness to handle this disorder. Our aim for this task is to curb our job around the MERS coronavirus and quick answer platforms to accelerate vaccine development.

"Our aspiration with that Technology would be to deliver a brand-new pathogen from gene order to clinical investigation in 16 months."

Other firms also working on Creating a vaccine comprise Janssen and Novavax; the latter Developed a vaccine from MERS.

In Addition, some businesses are exploring whether present anti-viral drugs Maybe successfully built to take care of this novel kind of coronavirus; a few Of them are drugs that have shown effectiveness against MERS and SARS previously. This strategy has been the main focus of this Australian Academy of Sciences; Researchers from the country happen to be testing 30 chemicals against 2019-nCoV.

CHAPTER THREE

Conspiracy of coronavirus

Two months later, China first reported that a deadly epidemic of a new kind of coronavirus, the subject continues to dominate headlines all over the world. The virus has infected more than 95,000 people in 79 countries and killed over 3,200.

The disease's rapid spread was accompanied by an epidemic of false promises and conspiracy theories on the societal and mainstream press, permitting misinformation about the roots of this virus and hoaxes on remedies to travel just as quickly as the disease.

One study from the US State Department, reported by the Washington Post, stated about 2 thousand tweets touting conspiracy theories regarding the virus - for example, claims it was brought on by a bioweapon - was published outside the US within the three-week period once the disease started to spread out China.

Based on Tedros Adhanom Ghebreyesus, head of the World Health Organization (WHO), these claims hamper the attempt to resist the COVID-19 epidemic.

"In WHO, we are not only battling the virus, but we are also fighting the trolls and conspiracy theorists that induce infantry and also sabotage the outbreak answer," he told reporters on February 8.

Stress, rumors, and bias

A bunch of 27 scientists in eight nations, including the US, Malaysia, and Australia, also condemned misinformation round the virus, even stating within an open letter on February 19 that conspiracy theories indicating COVID-19 doesn't have a natural source do "nothing but produce panic, rumors, and bias that jeopardize our worldwide alliance in the struggle against that virus."

Some analysts say its unsurprising false claims within the virus have thrived, largely since it's a new breed about that little is understood.

"An outbreak similar to this has lots of doubts, and if people do not have responses, and scientists aren't able to provide all of them of the replies and assurances they want, they're very likely to begin speculating," explained Marina Joubert, a mature science communicating researcher located in Stellenbosch, South Africa.

"Additionally, understandably, people are fearful and the pictures of individuals wearing masks and massive cities which are left-handed, cause additional stress," she added, speaking to lockdowns levied in a number of Italian and Chinese towns in an attempt to contain the epidemic.

Andrea Kitta, associate professor at East Carolina University in the united states, stated the "story patterns" of conspiracy theories surrounding the COVID-19 epidemic was indistinguishable to those in previous epidemics.

"In prior pandemics such as HIV or even H1N1, there were comparable conspiracy theories about bioengineering, plots to cull particular inhabitants, or that it is connected to sanitation and eating customs," she explained.

A widely circulated concept linked the virus into a movie of Chinese girl eating violin soup, that has been shared broadly on social networking and finally picked up by mainstream media websites including Russian social community, RT, along with British tabloid Daily Mail.

It later appeared that the clip was of a renowned Chinese vlogger ingesting the soup in Indonesia in 2016. While scientists consider bees are a distributor for the virus, they also suspect it might have jumped to people via a different creature host.

The bat soup assert is one of many accounts linking what Chinese men and women eat into the outbreak, and among many peddling racially charged asserts.

"A number of those stereotypes which have emerged would be that Chinese men and women are 'filthy' and they eat odd things. As soon as we do not have the info we are in need of, we have an inclination to speculate. However, sadly, that is where our inherent racism and prejudice begin to come in to play. We do so to allow ourselves to feel secure, but it is very problematic," explained Kitta.

Such claims could be harmful and have been connected to strikes and discrimination contrary to Chinese nationals and individuals of Asian origin in European nations like Italy and even against individuals evacuated from China from Ukraine.

What concerns some observers isn't merely misinformation about social websites, but some of those claims have forced their way to more mainstream outlets, such as in Saudi Arabia, Russia, and the United States.

From the first days of the epidemic, a columnist for popular Saudi paper al-Watan indicated on February 2 the new coronavirus had been a part of an attempt by Western pharmaceutical companies to gain by promoting vaccines for this, while the other columnist to the Syrian officer al-Thawra every day wrote on February 3 the virus had been a part of economic and mental warfare on China waged by the united states.

Similar claims have been aired on Russia's state-run Channel One. On February 5, a news anchor implied US President Donald

Trump was going to blame, linking the term corona, so crown Russian, to beauty pageants Trump was able to preside over.

In the united states, the right-wing press also has peddled conspiracy theories of their own, together with the Washington Times stating on January 24, the new coronavirus could have originated at a laboratory connected to China's "covert biological weapons program," a concept later endorsed by Republican Senator Tom Cotton.

Rush Limbaugh, a conservative radio host, stated the "coronavirus had been weaponized as another component to deliver down" Trump.

Geopolitics also played a part in the sort of misinformation being distributed, according to some analysts.

"Had the virus originated from a state not so important, it'd have been researched and found in another light," said Thitinan Pongsudhirak, a Thai political scientist and director of the Institute for Science and International Security, at Bangkok.

"China has problems with a lot of states, such as economic competition and behavioral tensions with the United States. It's dominant worldwide, and also Chinese tourists would be the most popular source for plenty of Asian nations. All this has influenced how in which the pandemic was reported."

An article in Foreign Policy magazine January 24 stated Chinese President Xi Jinping's"political schedule might prove to become a root cause for this outbreak," and his multibillion-dollar Belt along with Road Initiative has "made it feasible to get a neighborhood disease to develop into a worldwide menace."

'Bat soup along with bioengineering.'

Amid what WHO has become an "infodemic," societal networking firms have taken some actions to combat misinformation regarding the COVID-19 epidemic. Facebook, Twitter, and YouTube have announced steps to steer users searching for information about the coronavirus to credible resources, like the WHO.

But technology companies have to do more, " said Jonathan Corpus Ong, associate professor of international digital media at the University of Massachusetts Amherst in the United States.

"We are engaging for this health outbreak at another time from preceding outbreaks such as SARS or swine influenza. In the last several decades, a great deal of wellness disinformation and insidious fake information have been in a position to flourish online.

"This pandemic strikes us at the moment whenever there's far more rumor-mongering. Additionally, there are lots of social networking influencers who've been attempting to promote several types of merchandise. This is very hard to battle and fight," he explained.

"It is essential for conspiracy theories to be eliminated from online platforms earlier than was. Claims about bat soup along with bioengineering, as an instance, are still available," he explained. "Additionally, there has been too much attention on nudging to valid info and inadequate attention on shooting down hate addresses and slur."

Meanwhile, the pressure is also increasing on mainstream journalists to guarantee just and trustworthy coverage.

Joubert, the tech communicating researcher, stated: "I believe lots of the significant media businesses have done a fantastic job of supplying upgrades responsibly and to place experts ahead to talk to the general public. Regrettably, some smaller papers and radio channels could possibly be accountable for helping to spread misinformation."

She added: "The media must play a much larger part in making people conscious of misinformation and the reason it's essential to be crucial, and think logically if we absorb information, particularly in the internet world."

Conspiracy theorists blame the U.S. for coronavirus.

BEIJING -- The United States is hiding the real scale of its own coronavirus deaths. The United States must learn from China about how to react to an outbreak. The United States has been the source of this coronavirus -- along with the worldwide crisis wasn't China's fault.

As fresh coronavirus cases along with the feeling of fear ebb in China, the nation that was struck by the disorder was gripped by a wave of civic pride, conspiracy theories, and a recurrent mixture of anti-American thoughts: Proof, excellence, schadenfreude.

Weeks after China's government came under scrutiny whether its own mismanagement resisted the coronavirus around the Earth, officials at Beijing and lots of ordinary Chinese seem relieved -- happy -- to flip the tables and phone out missteps from Italy, South Korea and, especially, a Trump government that's been roiled with a disorderly response into the gathering catastrophe.

Lately, a run-of-the-mill mockery of this White House has taken a darker turn as the Chinese Web became overrun from the concept, subtly typified from the Chinese authorities, the coronavirus originated from the USA. Even the U.S. government, 1 variant of this concept goes, was covering mounting instances, and possibly tens of thousands of deaths, by substituting them as routine influenza.

While conspiracy theories pervade the Web in each nation, the abrupt surge and overwhelming incidence of anti-U.S. rhetoric that this week was conspicuous and important in the context of China, in which censors typically wash speech which strays from boundaries and authorities promptly detain those considered to be spreading rumors.

Coronavirus distributes from China. Now, China does not need to have the world dispersing it back again.

"Proceed WeChat, select Weibo, search on Baidu hunt, and it is filled with 'look at the rest of the states getting ill,' or 'the virus originated from the USA,' or all of the distinct heights of conspiracy theories," explained Xiao Qiang, an adjunct professor in the University of California in Berkeley's School of Information who researches China's Internet.

Fringe concepts, to be certain, have been broadly floated on each side of the Pacific.

Sen. Tom Cotton (R-Ark.) Theorized a month on Fox News, the virus could have escaped by a Wuhan laboratory that investigated harmful germs, repeating a favorite concept that was weathered by scientists.

A few observers of Chinese politics state the crescendo of anti-American sentiment could possibly be a commodity of natural nationalism or overactive imaginations of countless Chinese cooped up in the home. However, Xiao stated it was no denying that social websites -- the origin of information for many Chinese -- have been shrouded in anti-American discourse just at a time once the picture of the Communist Party and its chief Xi Jinping was badly dented following Chinese officials were discovered to be covering up ancient info regarding the epidemic.

"It is more than simply some disinformation or a formal story," said Xiao, the creator of China Digital Times, a site that regularly releases leaked directives in your party's propaganda division. "It is an orchestrated, all-purpose effort by the Chinese authorities through every station at a level that you seldom see. It Is a counteroffensive."

An overview of Chinese social networking and social media over recent times demonstrates how the anti-American notions obtained steam by means of a mixture of unexplained official announcements magnified by social networking, censorship, and doubts stoked by country media and police officers.

Zhong Nanshan, head of the China National Health Commission's group exploring the book coronavirus outbreak. (Thomas Suen/Reuters)

The frenzy turned into overdrive Feb. 27 following Zhong Nanshan, a Chinese pulmonologist that has emerged on state websites to provide crucial pronouncements, created a passing comment in a press conference, without providing any explanation that "the coronavirus first emerged in China but might never have originated in China."

Zhong's remarks were dismissed as exemplified by the respectable Shanghai public health officer Zhang Wenhong; nevertheless, Zhang's comments were immediately censored. Zhong later attempted to explain his remarks, but after that, nationalistic social networking reports and say media pounced.

State outlets started producing headlines that throw doubt on China's part in safeguarding the virus. China Global Television News, the international arm of the state broadcaster, uploaded a two-minute clip of Zhong's opinions to YouTube, garnering tens of thousands of viewpoints.

The rumor mill warms up. Influential Weibo accounts like "Beijing Matters" circulated a Taiwanese tv clip revealing a pharmacologist speculating concerning the United States since the contagion's origin. Writers at favorite sockets on WeChat churned out laying out the way the U.S. military might have set the pathogen as a covert bioweapon in a visit to Wuhan in October.

On Saturday, the New York-based College Daily, a favorite WeChat, accounts for Chinese students studying overseas that feet a nationalistic line-up, seen in a headline: "When it is correct that the virus originated from the USA if China nevertheless apologizes to the planet?"

When the broadly followed blogger Heiheig requested in a survey that afternoon, whether readers believed U.S. government information on influenza cases was questionable, 91% of the 116,000 respondents watched something fishy at U.S.-reported figures.

"They cannot fix covid-19so they are attempting to pin on China!" Said one common reaction. Others resisted the United States for not having the ability to create as many as sprays since China.

From Wednesday, Zhong's remarks came full circle. Foreign Ministry spokesman Zhao Lijian didn't speculate regarding the virus source or name some countries; however, he mentioned Zhong's remarks to conclude that China was not turned out to be the source.

"It is extremely reckless of a few media to predict the new coronavirus' native virus,'" and we strongly oppose it," Zhao told reporters in a daily briefing. "We must work together to combat the 'data virus' and the political climate. '"

Coronavirus checks Xi's'heavenly mandate,'" however reveals a godsend for his surveillance condition

The identical afternoon, the state-run Xinhua News Agency republished an article that indicated the virus originated, and that predicted for American journalists and officials to apologize.

Dali Yangan expert in Chinese politics at the University of Chicago stated he wasn't convinced that the outpouring of all anti-U.S. rhetoric was complete because of complicated state disinformation effort. However, the flood of articles and documents, lots of apparently written by real users, adapting together with the authorities' storyline that casts doubt on China's culpability, he explained.

"The objective is to decrease the focus on how China bungled its answer," explained Yang. "it is a type of blame-shifting."

Chinese beliefs and criticisms have never been restricted to the USA or black theories. Online posts have emerged from other authorities, from Italy to Japan.

A Chinese woman looks at her cell phone in the street in Beijing on Wednesday. (Kevin Frayer/AFP/Getty Images)

Bill Bishop, an author of Chinese politics that writes about the Sinocism publication, stated the story of Communist Party excellence has been -- and -- pushed. Following Hong Kong's pro-democracy protests, party leaders solved in November to double back on propaganda and also patriotic schooling that could tout the benefits of the celebration's effective, authoritarian leadership within disorderly, Western-style democracy," Bishop stated.

That debate is gaining traction," Bishop explained, adding his mother-in-law at China was advocating his family flee their home in Washington for the security of China.

"She's compelling us that China has won the virus conflict along with the U.S. is going to descend into madness," he explained.

It is uncertain how much the rhetoric bashing different nations will proceed. Most Chinese are expressing dismay at other people's online behavior.

An editorial writer in the China Youth Daily," Cao Lin, composed it was "gruesome" to watch Western "gloating over misfortune" and also "demonizing" other nations as the outbreak goes globally.

"It is belittling others' antivirus attempts to nourish pander for your sense of vanity," Cao wrote.

But unlike Cao, many others happen to be rapidly silenced for rebuking their own compatriots.

Wang Xiaolei, a former country media journalist and favorite WeChat essayist, urged the Chinese to quit blaming other nations and shoulder any responsibility.

Without scrutinizing the virus, Wang employed a very long sighting that contrasted China with renters whose flat flooding -- then attribute their own downstairs neighbor.

"Be an individual who has healthy psychology and fixes your flooring," Wang wrote in an article that has been criticized by powerful country press officials, such as Hu Xijinthe editor of the Global Times paper.

Coronavirus myths, scams and conspiracy theories that have gone viral
From the 2011 movie Contagion, which tells the story of a fast-moving virus crossing the planet, two personalities are particularly instructive.

There is Elizabeth "Beth" Emhoff, played by Gwyneth Paltrow of all Goop celebrity, with an affair at the wee hours of the epidemic and immediately dies. She's obviously unaware that many viruses, for example, coronavirus, are infections spread by droplets.

Then there is Alan Krumwiede; a mysterious conspiracy theorist played with Jude Law. He purchases into each fantasy circulating concerning the virus also helps regenerate them. In the end, he cries too, but not until his fake information effort has wiped out tens of thousands of other people.

We do not desire Telegraph readers following at the forefront of Beth or even Alan. Here are the very best tens scams and myths coursing the net, which you have to know about.

Jude Law's role from the 2011 movie Contagion -- conspiracy theorist Alan Krumwiede -- spreads information concerning treatment for the lethal virus CREDIT: Film Stills

1. Now you should be wary of getting bundles from China

FALSE. Regardless of what web conspiracy theorists could imply, it's safe to get an article from China. The World Health Organization has analyzed the length of viruses live on packages or letters and states those getting an email from China aren't in danger.

2. Cocaine can destroy the coronavirus

FALSE. The French tradition of health was made to scotch rumors that Bolivian marching powder could kill the virus following a run of bogus stories started circulating on the web. Red wine, Gauloises, along with a Gallic shrug, can also be regarded as ineffective.

3. Alcohol can ruin the coronavirus

FALSE. In a similar vein, booze won't stop you from catching the virus. Based on the official news agency, Irna, 16 individuals in Iran expired from methanol poisoning after drinking bootleg alcohol. When it's moonshine or even the best Merlot - the tipple of choice won't heal coronavirus.

4. Hand sprays kill the coronavirus

FALSE. No, not those produced with James Dyson! Hand dryers aren't helpful in eliminating the coronavirus or some other known virus. To safeguard yourself, wash your hands regularly using an impracticable hand wash or scrub them with water and soap. Once your hands have been washed, you must dry them completely using paper towels or some hot air drier.

5. Spraying chlorine and alcohol throughout your entire body will destroy the new coronavirus

FALSE. Doh! Spraying chlorine or alcohol throughout your body won't help. You aren't American poultry. "Spraying such compounds can be detrimental to garments or mucous membranes (i.e., eyes, mouth)"and warns that the WHO. "chlorine and alcoholism may be practical to disinfect surfaces, but they will need to get utilized under proper recommendations."

6. Drinking 'Miracle Mineral Remedy' will ruin the virus

FALSE. Followers of this pro-Trump Qanon conspiracy concept possess allegedly been encouraging other people to fight the coronavirus by ingesting a material called "Miracle Mineral Option."

The liquid includes bleach and has additionally been promoted as a miracle remedy for everything from pneumonia and HIV. Do not fall for this scam!

7. Eating garlic can help prevent disease with the new coronavirus

FALSE. Garlic can help ward off witches. however, it's useless against the coronavirus. It is a healthful food which could involve some antifungal qualities. But, there's "no evidence contrary to the present epidemic that ingesting garlic has shielded individuals from your brand-new coronavirus," says the WHO.

Empty plastic bottles created to makeshift full-face masks Won't protect you CREDIT: AFP

8. Coronavirus was leaked by a top security laboratory in Wuhan, and now China Is Attempting to cover up it

FALSE. About as possible as the Salisbury novichok assault of this past year derives from our very own high-security lab at Porton Down that isn't over a stone's throw away from the historical town. In summary, it is total nonsense up there with all wacko notions regarding 9/11, the Holocaust, and the death of JFK. The coronavirus is merely one more zoonotic disease - a virus that jumped from animals to people. Spanish influenza, HIV, and Ebola are the others.

9. Saline bleach and rinse can help stop the disease

FALSE. The bathroom cabinet isn't likely to supply any more aid in combating coronavirus compared to the kitchen cabinet (unless it's to recover soap or hand sanitizer). Regrettably, there's not any evidence to indicate that frequently draining the nose with either saline or saline mouthwash may ward off Covid-19.

10. Covering up using DIY masks and security Is a Great idea

FALSE. Today we're deeply in Alan Krumwiede land (see pic above). The internet is awash with pictures of people wearing everything from face masks created of fruit to airsoft helmets forged out of water bottles that are recycled. Elsewhere earnings of newspaper masks have gone through the roof. Do some of these preventative methods really work? No. Water bottles and plastic bags are worn across the head pose a possible suffocation hazard. Even surgical masks will probably not assist. They're made to maintain droplets inside, not outside, and need to be changed regularly.

11. All hand sanitizers may protect you from disease

FALSE. In the instance of hand sanitizers, maybe not all are created equal. They are incredibly helpful when commuting or traveling, and since they do not call for a constant visit into a spout that they are less difficult to make a custom of using often. However, in case your mobile cleaner comprises less than 60 percent alcohol -- or worse, not one -- it will not provide much protection in any way. Professional information in the PHE and the World Health Organization says that hand sanitizers should include at least 60 percent alcohol to be genuinely powerful.

CHAPTER FOUR

ANIMAL RELATED CORONAVIRUSES

The development of severe acute respiratory syndrome (SARS) exemplifies that coronaviruses (COVS) can quiescently emerge from potential animal reservoirs and may cause potentially deadly disease in people, as formerly known for creatures. Hence the focus of the review is going to be on the development of fresh COV strains as well as the relative pathogenesis of SARS COV with these COVS, which lead to enteric and respiratory ailments of different animal hosts. An overview of creature COV vaccines lately was published in media; therefore, this subject won't be dealt with.

The emergence of New Coronaviruses

The medical community has been astonished by the development of a new coronavirus associated with SARS in healthy adults in 2003. Historically individual COV diseases (229E and OC43 COV breeds) were moderate and correlated with just common cold symptoms even though reinfections, despite exactly the identical strain, happen. But, veterinary corona virologists had recognized the possibility of coronaviruses to induce deadly enteric or respiratory ailments in animals and to get brand new COV strains to originate out of unidentified reservoirs, frequently evoking deadly disorder in naïve inhabitants. As an instance, the porcine epidemic diarrhea COV (PEDV) first emerged from an unidentified origin in Europe and Asia from the 1970s and 1980s, resulting in acute diarrhea and prevalent deaths in baby pigs before getting embroiled in swine (Pensaert, 1999). The PEDV is headquartered in U.S. swine. Lately, PEDV is more closely linked to individual COV 229E compared to another creature category I COV (Duarte et al., 1994), also unlike another group that I COV, it develops in Vero cells such as SARS COV. These observations raise fascinating but unanswered questions regarding its source.

Or new COV strains Different in tissue tropism and virulence may come up from existing breeds. The virulent porcine respiratory coronavirus (PRCV) developed because of spike (S) gene deletion mutant of this exceptionally virulent enteric COV, transmissible gastroenteritis virus (TGEV). Curiously, differences between the dimensions of their 5′ finish S gene deletion area (621--681 nucleotides) between Western and U.S. PRCV breeds supplied evidence for their individual source on 2 continents in a similar timeframe (the 1980s). Deletion of the area (or in conjunction with deletions at ORF 3a) presumably accounted for modified tissue tropism from enteric to lymph and decreased virulence of their PRCV strains. The capability of particular COVS to persist within their host additionally provides a more chance for new mutants to be chosen with modified tissue tropisms and virulence from one of the viral RNA quasispecies (or a loaf of germs). A good instance is that the virulent systemic form, the feline infectious peritonitis virus (FIPV), that probably arises from chronic infection of cats using the virulent feline enteric COV.

Moreover, creature COVS may acquire New genes through recombination, according to the purchase of a flu C-like hemagglutinin by bovine COV or its ancestor COV. Recombination events among COVS can also produce new strains with the modified host or tissue tropisms. By way of instance, targeted recombination between mouse and feline S proteins empowers feline COV to infect mice (Haijema et al., 2003). Recent phylogenetic analysis indicates that SARS COV could have evolved in a previous recombination event involving mammalian-like along with avian-like parent breeds together with the S receptor symbolizing a mammalian (category 1) --avian origin mosaic. This recognition in which COVS may further evolve into a host people to obtain brand new tissue tropisms or virulence through mutations or recombination indicates that similar events might happen when SARS COV continues in humans.

Effect of Allergic Co-Infections on COV Diseases, Infection, and Slimming

Shipping Stress is known as a Multifactorial, polymicrobial respiratory disease complex at young mature feedlot cows with various facets exacerbating respiratory disorder, such as BCOV infections. Shipping fever may be precipitated by numerous viruses, independently or in combination, such as viruses, much like frequent human respiratory ailments (BCOV, bovine respiratory syncytial virus, parainfluenza-3 virus), bovine herpesvirus viruses and viruses effective at mediating immunosuppression (bovine viral diarrheavirus, etc.)). The transport of cattle long distances into feedlots, as well as the commingling of cows from several farms, generates physical pressures that conquer the creature's defense mechanisms and gives close touch because of exposure to new germs or breeds never previously encountered. Such variables are similar to the physiological strain of long plane trips with intimate contact among people from diverse areas of earth, each of which might play a part in improving a person's susceptibility to SARS. For transport fever, a number of factors (viruses(anxiety) permit commensal bacteria of the rectal tissues. To infect the lungs, resulting in fatal fibrinous pneumonia. Like PRCV or even SARS infections, it's likely that antibiotic therapy of these people with the huge discharge of bacterial lipopolysaccharides (LPS) could precipitate the induction of proinflammatory cytokines, which might further improve lung damage. By way of instance, hens infected with PRCV accompanied with a subclinical dose of E. coli LPS in 24 hours developed improved fever and much more acute respiratory disease in contrast to every agent. They reasoned that the consequences were probably mediated by the considerably enhanced rates of proinflammatory cytokines caused by the bacterial LPS. Thus, there's a need to analyze both LPS and lung cancer cytokine levels in SARS sufferers as potential mediators of the harshness of SARS. Compounds (Chlamydia spp.) They have already been isolated from SARS patients; however, their function in boosting the harshness of SARS is undefined.

Interactions between PRCV along with other Respiratory viruses can also parallel the prospect of parallel or pre-existing respiratory viral diseases to socialize with SARS COV (for instance, metapneumoviruses, flu, reoviruses, respiratory syncytial virus [RSV], OC43 or 229E COV). Sequential dual diseases of pigs using all the astrovirus (order Nidovirales, such as COV) PRRSV followed 10 times by PRCV considerably increased lung lesions and decreased weight gains in contrast to every virus independently. The double infections also contributed to more dinosaurs shedding PRCV nasally for a protracted period and astonishingly, into stool shedding of PRCV. The lung lesions detected resembled people in SARS sufferers.

Inoculated hens with PRCV followed closely in 2-3 times by swine flu A virus (SIV). They discovered that SIV lung titters were decreased from the dually in comparison to the infected algae, but paradoxically the lung lesions were much more intense at the dually infected algae. They declared that the elevated levels of IFN-alpha triggered by PRCV may mediate disturbance with SIV replication but might also give rise to the improved lung lesions. These studies have been highly pertinent to possible double infections with SARS COV and flu virus and possible remedies of SARS patients using IFN alpha.

Effect of Course (Aerosols) and Profession on COV Diseases

Experimental inoculation of monkeys Using PRCV strains revealed that management of PRCV from aerosol when compared with the oronasal route, or at greater doses, led to high virus titters drop and more shedding. In different studies, higher PRCV doses triggered the more acute respiratory disorder. Pigs awarded 108.5 TCID50 of PRCV had significantly more acute pneumonia and pneumonia compared to hens exposed by touch, and greater intranasal doses of a different PRCV breed (AR310) triggered moderate respiratory disorder whereas lower doses generated subclinical infections. By analogy, hospital processes that may potentially create aerosols or vulnerability to high initial dosages of SARS COV can improve SARS transmission or contribute to an improved respiratory disorder.

Effect of Therapy with Corticosteroids on COV Diseases of Animals

Corticosteroids have been known to cause Immunosuppression and cut back the quantities of CD4 and CD8 T cells and also particular cytokine levels. Many hospitalized SARS patients have been treated with steroids to decrease lung inflammation; however, there are no statistics to estimate the results of the treatment on virus lung or respiratory disorder. A recrudescence of BCOV fecal shedding was detected in one of four winter dysentery BCOV infected cows treated with dexamethasone. Likewise, the treatment of elderly monkeys with dexamethasone before the TGEV challenge resulted in profuse diarrhea and decreased lymphoproliferative responses in the treated tribes. These statistics raise problems for corticosteroid therapy of SARS patients linked to potential transient immunosuppression resulting in improved respiratory disorder or improved and protracted COV shedding (super spreaders). Alternately, corticosteroid treatment might be advantageous in reducing pro-inflammatory cytokines when discovered to play a significant part in lung immunopathology.

Group I Feline COV (FCOV): Model for Systemic and Continuous COV Infection

The range of disorder evident for FCOV (feline infectious peritonitis virus) illustrates the effects of viral persistence and macrophage tropism on COV disease severity and progression.

Historically, two sorts of FCOVS are known: feline enteric COV (FECOV) and FIPV. Present data suggest that the FECOV, which leads to acute enteric diseases in rodents, show persistent infections in certain cats, evolving to the systemic virulent FIPV in 5 to 10 percent of cats. The significance of the version to SARS is if comparable chronic COV infections may occur in certain patients, resulting in the development of macrophage-tropic mutants of improved virulence and precipitating systemic or immune-mediated disease. The first page of FCOV replication is from the pharyngeal, respiratory, or intestinal epithelial cells, and also clinical signs include anorexia, lethargy, and moderate diarrhoea. The protracted incubation interval for FIPV and its reactivation upon exposure to immunosuppressive viruses or corticosteroids implied that FCOVS might cause chronic enteric diseases. Recent reports of chronic fecal dropping and persistence of FCOV mRNA or antigen in infected moms affirm this situation.

A crucial pathogenetic occasion for Growth of FIPV is an effective infection of macrophages accompanied by cell-associated viremia and systemic dissemination of the virus. Anxiety (immunosuppressive ailments, transfer to new surroundings, cat density) resulting in immune suppression might cause FIP in chronically infected creatures, very similar to its function in transport fever COV diseases of cattle. Two main kinds of FIP happen: (1) effusive, using a fulminant course and passing within weeks to months, and (two) no effusive, progressing much more slowly. The effusive type is distinguished with fibrin-rich fluid accumulation in peritoneal, pleural, pericardial, or lymph areas, together with anorexia, fever, and weight reduction. No effusive FIP entails pyogranulomatous lesions together with thrombosis and central nervous system or ocular involvement. Fulminant FIP with hastened premature deaths seems to be resistantly evidenced in FCOV seropositive cats. At least 2 mechanisms implicating IgG antibodies to FCOV protein at FIP immunopathogenesis are clarified. At the very first, circulating immune complexes (IC) with C' depletion in sera and IC in lesions have been obvious from cats using terminal FIP. At the next, antibody-dependent enhancement (ADE) of FCOV infection of macrophages in vitro is mediated by neutralizing IgG MABS into the S protein FIPV, or of attention, into the antigenically-related COV, TGEV. A similar accelerated disorder was found in vivo in rodents inoculated with recombinant vaccinia virus expressing the alpha (although not the N or M proteins) of FIPV. Hence the FIPV version gives a terrifying glimpse of their seriousness and possible complications related to a chronic, systemic COV disease.

Group III COVS: Infectious Bronchitis Virus (IBV): Model for Bipolar COV Infection with Additional Target Tissues

The IBV is an Extremely infectious Respiratory disease of cows, such as SARS, spread by aerosol or maybe fecal-oral transmission, also spread globally. Genetically and antigenically closely associated COV are isolated out of pheasants and turkeys, but in young turkeys that they induce mostly enteritis. Respiratory diseases of cows are characterized by tracheal rales, coughing, and coughing, together with the disorder most acute in girls. The IBV also reproduces from the oviduct, inducing reduced egg production. Nephritogenic breeds can lead to mortality in young animals. In broilers, acute illness or death derives from systemic E. coli co-infection following IBV harm to the lymph nodes or Mycoplasma sp. Co-infections using IBV. The IBV is regained from the lymph nodes for approximately 28 days following infection and out of the feces following clinical recovery, together with all the cercal tonsil being a potential reservoir to IBV persistence, as the endurance of FCOV at the gut of cats. The IBV was retrieved in tracheal and cloacal swabs in cows at the start of egg production, indicating re-excretion of IBV from chronically infected birds, as well attested for mosquito reduction of FCOV or even BCOV later induction of immunosuppression.

The IBV reproduces in epithelial Cells of the trachea and bronchi, intestinal tract, oviduct kidney, and liver, resulting in necrosis and edema with little regions of pneumonia around large bronchi from the lymph nodes as well as interstitial nephritis from the gut. Of fascination with SARS is that the persistence of IBV from the liver as well as its protracted fecal shedding since SARS COV is found in urine and drop longer duration from feces. But it's unclear whether SARS COV dropping in urine is a result of viremia or even a kidney disease like IBV. Both identification and control of IBV are complex by the occurrence of numerous serotypes and the incidence of IBV recombinants. This is similar to the situation for many group 1 or two respiratory COVS, where just one or 2 (FCOV) serotypes have been understood. Also pertinent to SARS COV is that the discovering that IBV strains also replicate in Vero cells, but just after passing in chicken embryo cells.

In Conclusion, studies of creature COV Infections from the pure host supply enteric and respiratory disorder variations which improve our comprehension of the similarities and divergence of both COV disease pathogenesis and objectives for management. Unanswered queries for SARS pathogenesis, but highly pertinent to the style of plans for avoidance and management, comprise the following: what's the first site of viral replication? Why is SARS COV pneumonitis such as BCOV, with varying levels of disease of the respiratory and intestinal tracts and disorder characterized by the co-factors shared or unknown factors? Or, is SARS mostly targeted into the lung such as PRCV, together with mosquito reduction of swallowed virus and also with undefined sequelae leading to the diarrhea instances? Can SARS COV interrupt the lung directly or through viremia after the first replication in a different website (oral cavity (Fig (upper respiratory tract) also does this productively infect secondary target tissues (intestine, kidney) through viremia following replication in the gut?

Last, the constant, macrophage Tropic, systemic FIPV COV disease of cat's gifts still another COV disease Model and also a problem for tried control plans. This disease situation, the Induction of neutralizing IgG antibodies into the FIPV S protein, not simply neglects to avoid FIPV infections; however, it really potentiates the immunopathogenesis of FIPV.

The Suspected zoonotic source of SARS COV and the established propensity of many COV to cross species barriers exemplify the need for further animal research of the mechanics of interspecies transmission of COVS and adaptation into new hosts. The potential animal reservoir for SARS remains undefined. At present, we know very little about COVS or alternative germs circulating in wildlife or Their capability to emerge or recombine with present COVS (Starriness and also Guttman, 2004) an animal or public health dangers. Hopefully, the SARS outbreak Will create new interest and financing for these basic research queries Applicable not just on SARS COV, but in addition to this estimated 75% of recently Emerging human diseases originating as zoonoses.

CHAPTER FIVE
SPREAD OF CORONAVIRUS

Recent information suggests COVID-19 could possibly be passed from person to person. Additionally, there are a lot of unknowns, such as how infectious it may be.

The spread of the new coronavirus Is being tracked by the Centres for Disease Control (CDC), the World Health Organization, and wellness associations such as Johns Hopkins around the world. On Jan. 30, the World Health Organization announced that the COVID-19 epidemic a public health crisis.

How can this new coronavirus disperse to people?

COVID-19 emerged in Wuhan, a town In China, in December 2019. Though health officials are still tracing the precise origin of the new coronavirus, ancient hypotheses believed it could possibly be associated with a fish market in Wuhan, China. Some men and women who see the marketplace developed viral pneumonia resulting from the new coronavirus. A study that came out on Jan. 25, 2020, notes the person with the very first reported instance became sick about Dec. 1, 2019, and had no link to the fish marketplace. Investigations are continuing about how this virus originated and disperse.

This virus likely initially Emerged out of an animal origin but today appears to be spreading from person to person. COVID-19 was detected in people through China and 24 different nations, such as the USA.

What is the incubation time for COVID-19?

It Seems that symptoms are revealing Up in individuals inside 14 days of exposure to this virus.

What are the indications of COVID-19?

COVID-19 symptoms include:

· Cough

· Fever

· Shortness of breath

In rare cases, COVID-19 can result in Severe respiratory problems, kidney failure, or death.

If You've Got a fever or Any Sort of Respiratory problems like coughing or shortness of breath, call your health care provider or a healthcare provider and clarify your symptoms on the telephone prior to visiting the physician's office, urgent care center or emergency area.

On the telephone, Be Certain to inform them In case you've travelled outside the nation in the previous 14 days, especially to states influenced by COVID-19 (presently China, Iran, Italy, Japan, and South Korea). Moreover, make certain to inform them if you guess you've been near (within 6 feet) of somebody who gets COVID-19 for a protracted period. Your healthcare provider or your emergency room staff will recommend the following steps.

What's COVID-19 recognized?

Identification can be difficult using just A physical examination since moderate instances of COVID-19 may seem like the flu or a bad cold. A lab test may confirm the identification.

What's COVID-19 handled?

As of This Moment, There's not a certain Cure for the virus. Individuals who become ill from COVID-19 ought to be treated with supportive measures: people who alleviate symptoms. For acute cases, there can be additional alternatives for therapy, such as study medications and therapeutics.

Can COVID-19 induce death?

On Feb. 28, 2020," 2,871 deaths Have been credited to COVID-19. But, 36,687 individuals have recovered from this disease.

Can it be coronavirus distinct from SARS?

SARS Stands for severe acute respiratory disease. Back in 2003, an epidemic of SARS began in China and spread to several other nations before finishing in 2004. The virus, which leads to COVID-19, is much like the one which triggered the 2003 SARS epidemic: the two are forms of coronaviruses. Much remains unknown; however, COVID-19 appears to propagate quicker compared to the 2003 SARS and may cause less acute illness.

How can you protect yourself from this coronavirus?

Even the Centres for Disease Control and Prevention (CDC) has those Hints:

- Wash your hands regularly and thoroughly for 20 or more seconds. Use alcohol-based hand sanitizer if soap and water are not offered.
- Cover coughs and sneezes with a tissue, then throw the tissue from the garbage.

- Avoid touching your eyes, nose, or mouth with unwashed handsome.
- Stay home when You're sick.
- Clean and disinfect surfaces and items people often touch.

Which are the steps for coronavirus?

Many health bureaus in China and Other nations, such as the Centres for Disease Control (CDC) from the USA and the World Health Organization (WHO), are keeping a cautious eye with this disorder and taking measures to stop it from dispersing.

Timeline:

The World Health Organization (WHO) Has announced a global health crisis on a brand-new coronavirus, which causes a disease formally called COVID-19, which has murdered over 2,900 people globally.

Below is a deadline.

More:

Coronavirus: All you Want to know about the symptoms and dangers

How can coronavirus distribute, and how do you protect yourself?

Coronavirus: What nations have supported new scenarios?

On December 31 Final year, China Alerted WHO to many instances of odd pneumonia in Wuhan, a port city of 11 million people in the central Hubei province. The virus has been unknown.

A few of those contaminated functioned at the town's Huanan Seafood Wholesale Industry, which was closed down to January 1.

As health specialists worked to identify the virus amid rising alarm, the number of diseases exceeded 40.

On January 5, Chinese officials Ruled out the chance that this is really a recurrence of the severe acute respiratory syndrome (SARS) virus - a disease that originated in China and murdered over 770 people globally in 2002-2003.

On January 7, officials declared They'd identified a virus, according to the WHO. The publication virus has been called 2019-nCoV and has been recognized as belonging to the coronavirus family, which comprises SARS and the frequent cold.

Coronaviruses are common and also disperse Via being in proximity to a contaminated individual and inhaling droplets created if they cough or sneeze, or touching a face at which those droplets land then touching one's nose or face.

On January 11, China declared its First departure from the virus, even a 61-year-old guy who had bought goods from the fish marketplace. Therapy did not enhance his symptoms once he had been admitted into the hospital and that he died from heart failure on the night of January 9.

On January 13, the WHO reported that a Situation in Thailand, the first out of China, at a girl who had come from Wuhan.

On January 16," Japan's wellbeing Ministry reported that a confirmed case at a guy who had visited Wuhan.

But on January 17, as another departure was Documented in Wuhan, health officials from the US declared that the three airports might begin screening passengers coming from town.

Police in the USA, Nepal, France, Australia, Malaysia, Singapore, South Korea, Vietnam, and Taiwan supported instances within the next days.

On January 20, China reported that a Third departure and over 200 diseases, together with instances reported out Hubei state, including from the capital Beijing, Shanghai, and Shenzhen.

A Chinese specialist on Infectious diseases affirmed human-to-human transmission to say broadcaster CCTV, increasing fears of a significant outbreak as countless went for its Lunar New Year holiday.

Asian nations awakened steps to obstruct the spread of this virus, introducing compulsory screenings at airports of arrivals from high-risk regions of China.

On January 22, the death toll on China jumped into 17 with over 550 infections. Many European airports pop up tests on flights out of Wuhan.

Wuhan was put under effective Quarantine on January 23 as rail and air departures were also suspended.

The Very Same steps were announced for Two cities in Hubei state: Xiantao along with Chibi.

Beijing cancelled occasions for the Lunar New Year, beginning on January 25, while officials reported that the first death outside Hubei.

The WHO said in the future January 23, the epidemic didn't constitute a general emergency of worldwide concern and that there was "no proof" of this virus spreading between people beyond China.

Coronavirus

From January 24, the death toll on China stood at 26, with the authorities reporting over 830 infections.

The Number of towns under lockdown In Hubei climbed to 13, impacting 41 million individuals.

Shanghai Disneyland shut, and other Cities declared the close of entertainment places. Beijing stated a part of the Great Wall, along with other renowned landmarks, would likewise be shut.

On January 25, traveling limitations Were enforced on a further five towns in Hubei, carrying the general number of individuals changed to 56 million.

Hong Kong meanwhile announced a virus Emergency, cancelled Lunar New Year parties, and limited connections to southern China.

On January 26, the death toll climbed to 56, with nearly 2,000 cases supported as travel restrictions have been raised, and Hong Kong shut its Disneyland along with Ocean Park parks.

New cases were verified in the United States, Taiwan, Thailand, Japan, and South Korea.

On January 27, the death toll on China climbed to 106, with 100 in Hubei province, police reported. Another 4,515 individuals in China were reported to become infected. You will find 2,714 confirmed instances in Hubei province up from 1,423 the afternoon before.

On January 30, the WHO announced Coronavirus an international crisis since the death toll in China jumped into 170, together with 7,711 cases reported from the nation, in which the virus had spread to all 31 states.

India and the Philippines supported Their initial instances of this virus, together with a single infected individual in every nation.

On January 31, the Number of Confirmed cases in China jumped into 9,809. Russia, Spain, Sweden, and the United Kingdom confirmed its first cases of this virus.

On February 1, the death toll on China climbed to 259, together with 11,791 confirmed diseases in the nation, according to new statistics published by the Chinese health authorities.

New cases were verified in Australia, Canada, Germany, Japan, Singapore, the US, the UAE, and Vietnam.

On February 2, the very initial death Outside China, of a Chinese guy in Wuhan, has been reported from the Philippines.

The death toll in China climbed to 304, With 14,380 illnesses reported.

On February 3, China reported 57 brand new Deaths, bringing its death toll on 361. The number of cases rose to 17,205 around the nation.

On February 4, China stated the death Toll climbed to 425 individuals, and the number of infected individuals arrived at 20,438 at the mainland. Hong Kong also reported death, attracting international deaths to 427. The very first case has been confirmed in Belgium at someone who was repatriated out of Wuhan.

On February 5, longer flights Evacuating US citizens returned in Wuhan along with the WHO reaffirmed there was "no known successful remedy" for its coronavirus.

Meanwhile, China reported 490 deaths And 24,324 instances of disease.

On February 6, the death toll on Mainland China climbed to at least 563, with over 28,000 cases supported.

Meanwhile, police in Malaysia Reported that the nation's earliest known human-to-human transmission along with the range of individuals infected in Europe attained 30.

On February 7, Li Wenliang, a Physician Who was one of the first to sound the alert within the coronavirus, expired, also Hong Kong introduced prison sentences for anybody breaching rules.

Mainland China affirmed the departure Toll had attained at 636, together with 31,161 instances of disease, and Chinese researchers indicated the pangolin might have been a single connection in the series of animal-human ailments.

On February 8, a US taxpayer expired in Wuhan.

A Japanese guy in his 60s with a Suspected coronavirus disease also died in hospital at Wuhan, Japan's foreign ministry stated.

The death toll in China attained 722, With 34,546 affirmed infections.

China under stress as coronavirus Death toll surpasses SARS (3:22)

On February 9, the death toll on China surpassed the 2002-03 SARS outbreak, together with 811 deaths listed and 37,198 ailments.

An investigative team headed by specialists In the WHO left for China.

On February 10, China had 908 Confirmed deaths, and a total of 40,171 ailments - 97 brand new deaths have been reported after the most bizarre day of this epidemic.

President Xi Jinping seemed in People for the very first time since the outbreak started, seeing a hospital in Beijing and advocating optimism in the struggle against this virus.

On February 11, the WHO declared the new coronavirus would be known as"COVID-19".

Meanwhile, the deaths in China attained 1,016, together with 42,638 ailments listed.

On February 12, you will find 175 Individuals infected board the Diamond Princess cruise boat, docked at Yokohama, the Japanese health ministry stated.

The death toll from southern China struck 1,113, together with 44,653 ailments listed.

On February 13, North Korea levied A month-long quarantine on all overseas visitors, and many others supposed to get COVID-19, the Korean Central News Agency said.

The death toll from southern China struck 1,300, with almost 60,000 infections listed. Meanwhile, Japan confirmed its first departure from the virus.

On February 14, Egypt became a First country in Africa to record that a situation and France reported Europe's first departure from the virus.

China reported 121 further deaths. Bringing into the entire amount throughout the mainland to almost 1,400.

February 15 watched the death toll on Mainland China surge beyond 1,500, together with 66,492 diseases confirmed in southern China.

Elsewhere, the United States ready to Evacuate its citizens out of a cruise boat quarantined in a Japanese pier.

Meanwhile, a February 3 address by Chinese President Xi Jinping, released by state media, also suggested the authorities knew about the danger of this virus well prior to the public alert was increased.

CARD: Coronavirus deadline

On February 16, Taiwan listed its First departure of a cab driver at his 60s on account of this coronavirus.

Authorities noted that 1,665 People had perished in southern China, with 68,500 instances of the disease reported.

On February 17, you will find 1,770 Deaths reported in southern China and 70,548 instances.

Japan supported 99 new Instances of this Virus board that the quarantined Diamond Princess cruise boat.

February 18 watched China's daily Disease figures fall below 2,000 for the first time since January, together with the nation's health commission coverage 72,436 ailments over the mainland and 1,868 deaths.

Meanwhile, Russia said it might prohibit Entrance for Chinese citizens from February 20.

Coronavirus outbreak: Ethiopia measures Up avoidance steps (2:50)

On February 19, Iran reported just two Deaths in the coronavirus, hours later confirming its initial circumstances.

China's daily disease figures fall Under 2,000 for the 2nd consecutive day, together with the nation's health commission coverage 74,185 ailments over the mainland and 2,004 deaths.

On February 20, South Korea reported Its first departure from the coronavirus.

Meanwhile, China reported that the death toll had climbed to 2,118, while the whole number of cases attained 74,576. The nation's health commission reported everyday illnesses fell to the bottom in nearly a month, as a consequence of government only counting instances supported by genetic testing in Hubei.

On February 21, South Korea reported Its second departure and 100 brand new confirmed cases of this coronavirus, bringing the total to 204. In southern China, the death toll reached 2,236 since the verified cases of the disease improved above 75,400.

Additionally, Israel reported its original Confirmed instance of this coronavirus following a girl who returned from a cruise boat tested positive.

Back in Italy, the region of Lombardy Reported that the first community transmission of this virus using three new instances, bringing the total from the state to six illnesses.

South Korea: Emergency steps Later increase in coronavirus instances (1:59)

On February 22, South Korea saw its own Biggest spike in one day using 229 new instances of this virus.

Italy reported its initial two deaths, While Iran affirmed a fifth death, one of 10 new illnesses. A sixth departure was afterward verified, although it wasn't clear if this instance was contained in the nation's 28 confirmed cases.

In southern China, the Number of new Infections dropped considerably, with 397 instances reported.

February 23 saw a few Nations Near their borders with Iran because the number of diseases and deaths from the nation grew.

Back in Italy, officials affirmed the Third departure, while local governments introduced the Venice Carnival into an early closure and suspended sports occasions in an effort to fight the spread of this virus from Europe's worst-hit nation.

On February 24, Kuwait, Bahrain, Iraq, Afghanistan, and Oman reported that their first cases of this virus. Meanwhile, the number of cases at South Korea ballooned to 833 cases with seven deaths.

The death toll in China climbed to 2,595, one of 77,262 supported instances.

A death premiered in Northern Italy.

On February 25," Iran's deputy health Marriage, that had a day before giving a media briefing about the epidemic, affirmed he had coronavirus. The nation's official complete attained 95 instances with 15 deaths.

Meanwhile, China's reported instances Continued to innovate, with 518 fresh ailments and 71 fresh deaths verified. South Korea's confirmed cases climbed to 977 while Italy's attained 229.

On February 26, the international death Toll neared 2,800, using a total of roughly 80,000 confirmed disease cases reported worldwide.

Norway, Romania, Greece, Georgia, Pakistan, North Macedonia, and Brazil all discovered their very first instances of this coronavirus.

On February 27, Estonia, Denmark, Northern Ireland, and the Netherlands reported their very first coronavirus instances. The number of ailments passed 82,000 globally, including over 2,800 deaths.

Italy has witnessed a spike in diseases, which jumped into 650, while more people died with all the tally of dead individuals currently at 17.

Meanwhile, in America, the Government is considering devoting the Défense Production Act that will give President Donald Trump that the capability to enlarge industrial production of important substances or goods for national safety.

On February 28, Lithuania and Wales Reported their very first coronavirus instances, together with the Netherlands and also Georgia reporting their instant.

February 29 watched South Korea report Its greatest daily amount of verified cases nevertheless, 813, bringing the nation's total to 3,150 with 17 deaths. Iran reported the number of its instances had jumped 388 instances to 593 at 24 hours, together with all the death toll hitting 43.

What is the passing rate from COVID-19?

The biggest study on COVID-19 instances to date offers new details about the intensity of this disease, for example, its passing rate, and that is most vulnerable.

The study investigators, by the Chinese Center for Disease Control and Prevention, examined advice from 44,672 confirmed instances of COVID-19 from China, which has been reported between Dec. 31, 2019, and Feb. 11, 2020. In one of these situations, there have been 1,023 deaths, leading to a general passing rate of 2.3 percent.

That is Greater than the passing Speed of influenza, which can be approximately 0.1percent at the U.S., But, the new study revealed that the departure rate from COVID-19 varied from the place. Back in Hubei Province, where the epidemic started, the passing rate was 2.9%, in comparison to only 0.4percent in different countries -- a 7-fold gap.

The analysis also revealed that elderly Adults are hit hardest by COVID-19. One of those ages 80 and older, the passing rate was 14.8 percent, compared to 8.0percent for people ages 70 to 79; 3.6percent for people ages 60 to 69; 1.3percent for people ages 50 to 59; 0.4percent for people ages 40 to 49, and 0.2percent for people ages 10 to 39. No deaths have been reported among children from birth to age 9.

But some specialists have estimated That the amount of COVID-19 cases might be higher than that which was formally monitored and documented, according to the BBC. If that is the situation, then the death rate might be lower than what's documented in this research.

Why did coronavirus cases spike?

On Feb. 12, the Hubei Province, Where the epidemic started in Wuhan, officials have opted to think about a "clinical" diagnosis for the new coronavirus. That usually means these people who might have tested negative about the present diagnostic evaluation (known as a lipoic acid test) but reveal all the coronavirus symptoms will probably be categorized as confirmed instances. In this manner, the Hubei Province Health Committee explained, "patients may get standardized therapy based on verified cases as soon as you can to further enhance the success rate of therapy."

With this new standard, the state Additional 14,840 instances of coronavirus into the total a day.

Will the coronavirus expire down from the Summertime?

We do not understand yet. Most respiratory Viruses, like influenza viruses, are somewhat seasonal. We normally understand when the peak of influenza season will soon be and will anticipate the number of influenza cases to fall down as we go toward summer and spring, stated Dr. Nancy Meissonier, the director of CDC's National Centre for Immunization and Respiratory Diseases at a press conference on Feb. 12. However, for the virus, "that I think that it's premature to presume," she explained. If this virus acts similarly to influenza viruses, we might see fewer illnesses because spring and summer roll around. "But this really is a new disorder, we have not been through six months of it less per year," Meissonier explained. Though trusting the numbers will return as hot weather systems, "the competitive actions we are taking are since we do not believe we could count on this."

Who'll likely be quarantined in the USA?

Officials declared on Friday (Jan. 31) the U.S. would be implementing quarantines on taxpayers who have travelled into the Hubei Province (where the epidemic originated) in the previous 14 days. In case U.S. citizens have already been to China from the previous 14 days, they'll be rerouted to a few of eleven divisions throughout the nation to be screened to its new coronavirus, as stated by the Department of Homeland Security (DHS).

If passengers that have travelled to China are displaying signs of this virus (including a cough, difficulty breathing, or fever), they'll be subject to compulsory quarantines. If passengers that have visited China (out of their Hubei province) reveal no indications after being screened in a few of the 11 airports, then they'll be re-booked for their destinations over the U.S. and requested to self-quarantine in house, according to the DHS.

Other travellers that have not been to China, however, are discovered to be on precisely the exact same flight of passengers which were to China may likewise be transported to a few of those 11 airports, according to the DHS. What is more, generally, "foreign nationals" who've travelled to China from the previous 14 days will not be permitted from the U.S.

Countless U.S. citizens that were Evacuated from Wuhan and also even the Diamond Princess cruise boat were also put under compulsory quarantine at a few U.S. military foundations.

Does the coronavirus possess an Official title?

On Feb. 11," WHO Director-General Tedros Adhanom Ghebreyesus declared the official title of this new disease brought on by the publication coronavirus: Corona Virus Disease, called COVID-19. "Using a title thing to protect against using different titles which could be incorrect or stigmatizing. Additionally, it provides us a normal structure to use for any upcoming coronavirus outbreaks," Ghebreyesus explained.

WHO discourages planting fresh viruses After geographical locations, individuals, species, or groups of animals or meals, according to the business's Best Practices such as the Naming of New Human Infectious Diseases? Instead, WHO promotes the use of descriptive conditions of a disorder, for example, "respiratory illness" and also "bronchial syndrome," and "acute" or "progressive." The company also states that when a pathogen is understood, it needs to be utilized as a member of their disorder's name.

Where Did the new coronavirus come out of?

Since the virus popped up in Wuhan in people who had seen neighborhood seafood and creature market (known as the Huanan fish marketplace), officials might just say it probably hopped from a creature to people. In a new analysis, nevertheless, the researchers in comparison SARS-CoV-2 (previously 2019-nCoV) genetic arrangement together with people in a variety of viral sequences, also discovered the most closely associated viruses were just two coronaviruses which originated from rodents; the two of these coronaviruses shared 88 percent of the genetic arrangement by that of SARS-CoV-2.

Based on these outcomes, the authors Stated the SARS-CoV-2 probably originated in rodents. But no bats were offered in the Huanan fish marketplace, which implies another yet-to-be-identified animal functioned as a steppingstone of types to carry the virus into people.

A Minimum of One study has indicated. This "intermediate" creature has been the pangolin, a compromised, ant-eating mammal. But, complete data from this research hasn't yet been published, which makes the results difficult to confirm, as stated by the BBC.

A previous study indicated snakes, which were offered in the Huanan fish marketplace, as a potential supply of the virus that was new. But some specialists have criticized the study, saying it is uncertain if coronaviruses could infect bees.

How Does the coronavirus spread between individuals?

Scientists are still working to Know precisely how SARS-CoV-2 spreads. However, generally speaking, the most frequent method coronaviruses spread is via respiratory droplets generated from coughs and sneezes, according to the CDC. Tests also have discovered that the virus within patients' feces, implying it could possibly have the ability to propagate through fecal contamination. But, it's still uncertain whether people may catch the virus from touching surfaces that are contaminated, the CDC states.

The number of deaths from coronavirus has happened outside mainland China.

On Feb. 27, there were 69 reported deaths in the new coronavirus out of China. These include 26 deaths in Iran, 13 deaths in South Korea, 17 deaths in Italy, 4 deaths amongst passengers that have been aboard the Diamond Princess cruise boat, two deaths in Hong Kong, 3 deaths in Japan, two in France, and one each in Taiwan and the Philippines, according to Johns Hopkins University.

Could This virus trigger a pandemic?

Folks wear face masks as they wait In Hankou Railway Station on Jan. 22, 2020, at Wuhan, China, in which the new coronavirus 2019-nCoV originated.

For this particular virus, or even some other, to Cause a pandemic in people, it should do three things: effectively infect people, replicate in people then spread readily among people, Live Science formerly mentioned.

To Ascertain how readily the virus Spreads, scientists need to calculate what is called the "basic reproduction number, or even R_0 (conspicuous R-nought.) That is an indicator of the typical amount of folks that catch the virus in one infected individual, Live science formerly mentioned. A study released Jan. 29 at the New England Journal of Medicine (NEJM) estimated that an R_0 significance for its brand-new coronavirus to become 2.2, meaning every infected individual was spreading the virus into a mean of 2.2 people. This is very similar to previous estimates, which were put the R_0 worth between 3 and 2. (By contrast, SARS originally had an R_0 of approximately 3, until public health steps introduced it down to over 1)

Generally, a virus will probably continue to spread if it's an R-value of higher than 1, and consequently general health measures to Stem the outbreak should target to decrease R0 to less than you, the writers of this NEJM paper stated.

On Jan. 30, the World Health Organization (WHO) announced that the new coronavirus Outbreak is really a public health emergency of global concern. The primary reason for the announcement is concern that the virus may spread to nations with Weaker health programs.

How Can coronavirus compare to SARS and MERS?

A highly magnified image of this Middle East Respiratory Syndrome Coronavirus (MERS-COV). (Picture credit: CDC/Cynthia Goldsmith, Azaibi Taemin)

On Feb. 9, more people had expired in the new coronavirus compared to SARS -- that killed 774 individuals globally, according to The New York Times.

MERS and SARS have been known to cause acute symptoms in people. It is uncertain how a new coronavirus will evaluate in seriousness, as it's generated acute symptoms and death in many individuals while causing only mild illness from other people, according to the CDC. All three of those coronaviruses could be transmitted between people through contact.

MERS that was sent from Touching infected camels or swallowing their milk or meat has been initially reported in 2012 from Saudi Arabia and has largely been included from the Arabian Peninsula, based on NPR. SARS was first reported in 2002 in southern China (no new instances are reported since 2004) and can be considered to have spread from bats that infected civets. The new coronavirus was probably transmitted from eating or touching an infected creature in Wuhan.

Throughout the SARS outbreak, the virus Murdered roughly 1 in 10 individuals who had been infected. The passing rate from COVID-19 is anticipated to be a bit more than 2%.

Nevertheless, in the Start of an epidemic, The first cases which are recognized "skew into the acute," which can produce the mortality rate look higher than it's, Alex Azar, secretary of the U.S. Department of Health and Homeland Security (HHS), said during a news briefing on Tuesday (Jan. 28). The mortality rate could fall as more moderate cases are recognized, Azar said.

Presently, the Majority of the patients that Have died from the disease happen to be older than 60 and have had pre-existing ailments.

Do you know the signs of this new Coronavirus, and how can you cure it?

A thermometer. (Picture credit: Shutterstock)

Indicators of this new coronavirus Include cough, fever, and trouble breathing, according to the CDC. It is projected that symptoms might appear when two weeks or as long as 14 days following exposure, the CDC stated. The NEJM study printed on Jan. 29 estimated, normally, folks show symptoms about 5 times when they are infected.

There are no specific remedies for Coronavirus infections, and the majority of individuals will recover by themselves, according to the CDC. So, therapy involves rest and medicine to ease symptoms. A humidifier or warm tub can help relieve a sore throat and cough. If you're mildly ill, then you need to drink a lot of fluids and break, but if you're concerned about your symptoms, then you need to visit a physician, they composed. (This is information for many coronaviruses, not especially geared toward the virus).

On Feb. 25, U.S. officials declared The very first clinical trial in the nation to rate a remedy for COVID-19 had been penalized, according to the NIH. The trial will examine an antiviral medication known as remdesivir in elderly adults using COVID-19. The very first study manager is the American who caught the illness whilst onboard the Diamond Princess cruise ship and is now being treated at the University of Nebraska Medical Center (UNMC). The analysis could be adapted to analyze different treatments and register patients on other websites from the U.S. and worldwide, officials explained.

There's no vaccine to the new Coronavirus; however, researchers in the U.S. National Institutes of Health verified they were at preliminary phases of building one. Officials intend to establish a phase 1 clinical trial of a possible vaccine over the upcoming few weeks.

CHAPTER SIX
CORONAVIRUS SYMPTOMS AND CURE

Covering your mouth when coughing may Help block the spread of coronaviruses.

Researchers first circulated a coronavirus in 1937. They discovered a Coronavirus in charge of infectious bronchitis virus birds, which had the capability to devastate poultry shares.

Scientists first found evidence of Individual coronaviruses (HCoV) from the 1960s in the wake of individuals with the frequent cold. Two individual coronaviruses are accountable for a huge percentage of common migraines: OC43 and 229E.

The title "coronavirus" stems from That the crown-like projections onto their surfaces. "Corona" in Latin means "halo" or "crown."

Among people, coronavirus infections Most often happen during winter and premature spring. Folks often become sick with a cold because of a coronavirus and might catch the exact same one about 4 weeks later.

That is only because coronavirus Compounds don't endure for quite a very long moment. Additionally, the antibodies for a single strain of coronavirus might be ineffective against a different one.

Infection

Cold- or flu-like symptoms generally Put in from two --4 times following a coronavirus disease and therefore are normally mild. However, symptoms differ from person-to-person, and also a few types of this virus can be deadly.

Symptoms comprise:

- Infection
- runny nose
- tiredness
- Infection
- fever in rare instances
- sore throat
- exacerbated Infection

Scientists Can't easily nurture Human coronaviruses from the lab, unlike the rhinovirus, which can be another reason for the frequent cold. This makes it challenging to estimate the effects of the coronavirus on domestic markets and public health.

There's no cure; therefore, remedies Include over-the-counter and reflexology (OTC) medicine. Folks can take a few measures, such as:

- resting and preventing overexertion
- drinking sufficient water
- preventing smoky and smoking spots
- taking acetaminophen, aspirin, or naproxen for fever and pain
- Employing a sterile humidifier or cool mist vaporizer

A Physician may diagnose the virus Accountable for using a sample of lymph fluids, such as mucus in the nose, or even bloodstream.

Forms

Coronaviruses belong to the Subfamily Coronavirinae at the household Coronaviridae.

Various Kinds of human Coronaviruses change in how intense the consequent disease becomes, and also just how far they could disperse.

Doctors now recognize seven Kinds of coronavirus that could infect people.

Common forms Comprise:

- 229E (alpha coronavirus)
- NL63 (alpha coronavirus)
- OC43 (beta coronavirus)
- HKU1 (beta coronavirus)

Rarer breeds that cause more intense Complications comprise MERS-CoV, which induces Middle East respiratory disease (MERS), also SARS-CoV, the virus responsible for severe acute respiratory disease (SARS).

In 2019, a dangerous new breed Known as SARS-CoV-2 began circulating, inducing the illness COVID-19.

Transmission

Limited research is available on the way HCoV spreads from 1 individual to another.

However, researchers think that the viruses transmitted through fluids at the lymph tract, such as indigestion.

Coronaviruses can disperse in the Following manners:

- Coughing and sneezing without covering your mouth area could distribute droplets into the atmosphere.
- Touching or shaking hands with someone that has the virus may pass the virus involving people.
- Getting contact with a face or thing with the virus and then touching the nose, eyes, eyes, or mouth area.
- Some animal coronaviruses, like feline coronavirus (FCOV), can propagate through touch with stool. But, it's unclear if this applies to individual coronaviruses.

The National Institutes of Health (NIH) imply that many groups of individuals possess the highest risk of developing complications because of COVID-19. These classes comprise:

- young kids
- individuals aged 65 Decades or old
- girls That Are pregnant

Coronaviruses will sabotage most Individuals at any point during the course of their life.

Coronaviruses can mutate Effectively, making them so infectious.

To stop transmission, folks Should remain at home and break while symptoms are busy. They must also avoid contact with other individuals.

Covering your mouth and nose using a Tissue or handkerchief whilst coughing or coughing can also assist in preventing transmission. It's crucial to eliminate any cells after usage and keep hygiene around your house.

COVID-19

In 2019, the Centers for Disease Control and Prevention (CDC) began tracking the epidemic of a new coronavirus, SARS-CoV-2, which results in respiratory disease now called COVID-19. Authorities first recognized the virus at Wuhan, China.

Over 74,000 individuals have contracted the virus from China. Health Governments have identified a number of different individuals with COVID-19 across the planet, such as many in the USA. On January 31, 2020the virus passed from 1 individual to another from the U.S.

The World Health Organization (WHO) Has announced a public health crisis concerning COVID-19.

Since That Time, this breed was Diagnosed in many U.S. inhabitants. The CDC has suggested that it's possible to disperse many individuals. COVID-19 has begun causing a disturbance in 25 other nations.

The Very First people with COVID-19'd Linked into a creature and fish marketplace. This fact indicated that animals originally transmitted the virus to people. But, individuals with a more recent analysis had no relations or exposure to the current market, confirming that individuals could pass the virus to one another.

Advice on the virus would be rare at present. In earlier times, respiratory ailments that come from coronaviruses, like SARS and MERS, have dispersed through intimate contacts.

SARS

SARS was an infectious disease that Developed the following disease by the SARS-CoV coronavirus. Normally, it resulted in a life-threatening form of pneumonia.

During November 2002the virus Began at the Guangdong Province in southern China, finally attaining Hong Kong. From that point, it quickly spread across the Earth, causing diseases in over 24 nations.

SARS-CoV can infect the top and lower respiratory tracts.

The Signs of SARS grow over the span of a week and then begin with a fever. Early in the illness, individuals grow flu-like symptoms, for example:

· Dry coughing

· chills

· Infection

· breathlessness

· aches

Pneumonia, a serious lung disease, usually develops. At its most complex stage, SARS induces the collapse of their lungs, heart, or liver disease.

According to the CDC, police Marked 8,098 individuals as having contracted SARS. Of these, 774 diseases were deadly. This equates to a mortality rate of 9.6 percent.

Complications were more inclined in Older adults, and half of the people over 65 decades old who became sick didn't endure. Authorities finally commanded SARS in July 2003.

MERS

MERS spread as a Result of coronavirus Called MERS-CoV. Scientists recognized this acute respiratory disease in 2012; later, it surfaced from Saudi Arabia. Ever since that time, it's spread into other nations.

The virus has attained the U.S., While the biggest outbreak beyond the Arabian Peninsula happened in South Korea in 2015.

Indicators of MERS include Stress, and breathlessness, and coughing. The disease spreads through intimate contact with individuals who have an illness. But all instances of MERS have hyperlinks to people recently returning from traveling to the Arabian Peninsula.

What signs of being on the lookout for and the best way to protect yourself from coronavirus

What are the Indicators

Coronavirus makes people ill, and Usually using a moderate to moderate upper respiratory tract disease, very similar to a frequent cold. Its symptoms include a runny nose, cough, and sore throat, pain, and a fever that could last for a few days.

For Anyone with a diminished immune system, both the elderly and the very young, there is a possibility the virus may cause a lesser, plus far more severe, respiratory tract diseases such as pneumonia or pneumonia.

How Does it disperse

Transmission between people happens Whenever someone comes to contact with the infected person's secretions, like droplets at a cough.

Based on how virulent the virus Isa cough, sneeze, or the clot may lead to exposure. The virus may also be transmitted by coming in contact with something that an infected person has touched and after touching your mouth, eyes, or nose. Caregivers can, at times, be subjected by managing an individual's waste, according to the CDC.

The virus seems to mostly spread From person to person.

"Folks are thought to be Contagious when they're symptomatic (that the sickest). "Some disperse may be possible before individuals show signs; there were reports of this happening with... coronavirus; however, this isn't believed to be the principal way that the virus spreads."

How Might it be treated

There Is Not Any specific antiviral Treatment; however, research is still underway.

The Majority of the time, symptoms can proceed Off by themselves and pros counsel searching care early. If symptoms feel much worse compared to a typical cold, see your physician. Doctors may alleviate symptoms by means of a fever or pain medicine. The CDC claims that a room humidifier or even a hot shower can assist with a sore throat or cough.

Individuals with coronavirus ought to Receive supportive services to help alleviate symptoms. In certain severe cases, therapy includes a caution to encourage critical organ purposes, the CDC states.

Individuals that think they Might Have been Exposed to this virus must contact their healthcare provider promptly.

How Long is the incubation interval?

Quarantine is generally set up for your own Incubation period -- that the length of time through which individuals have grown sickness after exposure. To get coronavirus, the amount of quarantine is 14 days in the last period of vulnerability, since 14 days will be the longest incubation phase seen for comparable illnesses.

How Can you stop it?

There's no vaccine to protect Contrary to, at least not yet.

The US National Institutes of Health Is working in a vaccine, but it's going to be months before clinical trials have underway and over a year till it may become accessible.

Meanwhile, You Might Be able to decrease Your risk of disease by preventing people that are ill. Cover your nose and mouth when you cough or sneeze, and then purge the surfaces and objects that you touch.

Avoid touching your eyes, nose, and mouth. Clean your hands frequently with soap and warm water for a minimum of 20 minutes.

Awareness can also be crucial. If You're Ill and also have reason to think it might be more coronavirus, you need to let a healthcare provider understand and seek treatment early.

Reasons

It is uncertain exactly how infectious the brand-new coronavirus is. It seems to be spreading from person to person, one of those in contact. It could possibly be spread by respiratory droplets discharged when somebody using the virus coughs or sneezes.

Risk variables

Risk factors for COVID-19 seem to Comprise:

- Present traveling from or home in China
- Close contact with somebody who has COVID-19 -- like when a relative or healthcare worker handles an infected individual

Prevention

Although there's no vaccine available to avoid disease with the new coronavirus, it is possible to take action to lessen your chance of disease. WHO and CDC advocate following conventional precautions for preventing respiratory infections:

- Wash your hands frequently using soap and warm water, or even utilize a supplementary hand sanitizer.
- Cover your nose and mouth with your elbow or tissue whenever you sneeze or cough.
- Avoid touching your eyes, mouth, and nose if your hands are not clean.
- Avoid close contact with anyone who's sick.
- Prevent sharing meals, glasses, bedding, and other household things if you are sick.
- Wipe and clean surfaces that you frequently touch.
- Stay home from work, college, and public places if you are sick.

CDC does not recommend that healthy People today put on a facemask to protect themselves from respiratory disorders, such as COVID-19. Only put on a mask in case a healthcare provider tells you to do so.

WHO also recommends that you:

- Avoid eating uncooked or undercooked meat or animal organs.

- Prevent contact with live critters and surfaces they might have touched in case you see live niches in regions that have recently had new coronavirus instances.

Traveling

If you intend to travel Globally, first assess travel advisories. You might also need to speak to your health care provider when you have health issues that make you more vulnerable to respiratory complications and infections.

CHAPTER SEVEN
KEYS TO DIAGNOSIS, TREATMENT, AND PREVENTION OF SARS

For coronavirus researchers, the Recognition of a new coronavirus as the reason for the severe acute respiratory syndrome (SARS) was definitely impressive, yet not surprising. The cadre of researchers that have worked on this fascinating family of viruses within the last 30 years is conversant with lots of the qualities of coronavirus biology, pathogenesis, and disorder that triggered so radically in the global SARS outbreak. Advances in the biology of coronaviruses have led to greater comprehension of their ability for adaptation to new surroundings, transspecies disease, and the development of new diseases. New tools of molecular and cell biology have contributed to greater comprehension of intracellular replication and viral cell biology, as well as the introduction in the previous five decades of reverse genetic methods to research coronaviruses have made it feasible to start to identify the determinants of viral replication, transparencies adaptation, and human disorder. This short article will examine the fundamental life span and replication of this well-studied coronavirus, mouse hepatitis virus (MHV), identifying the distinctive features of coronavirus research, and highlighting crucial points where analysis has made important improvements, and which may represent goals for antivirals or pathogens. Regions, where rapid advancement was produced in

SCoV analysis, will be clarified. At length, areas of demand for study at coronavirus replication, genetics, and pathogenesis is going to be outlined.

Coronavirus Life Cycle

The very best-studied model for Coronavirus replication and pathogenesis has long become the group two murine coronavirus, mouse hepatitis virus, along with a lot of what's understood of the phases of this coronavirus life cycle was discovered in animals and also in civilization employing this particular virus. Hence this discussion will revolve around MHV with comparisons to both SCoV along with other coronaviruses. That is appropriate since bioinformatics investigations imply that SCoV, even though a different virus, contains important similarities in business, putative protein acts, and replication into the group II coronaviruses, especially within the replicase gene. Excellent, comprehensive testimonials of MHV and coronavirus replication can be found everywhere.

The coronavirus virion is an Enveloped particle comprising the spike (S), membrane (M), and envelope (E) proteins.) Additionally, some breeds of coronaviruses, although maybe not SCoV, say a hemagglutinin protein (HE), which can also be integrated from the virion. The genome of all coronaviruses is a terminal, single-stranded RNA molecule of favorable (mRNA) polarity, also by 28 to 32 kb in length. Inside the virion, the genome is encapsidated by numerous duplicates of the nucleocapsid protein (N), also contains the conformation of a helical RNA/nucleocapsid construction. The protein was a focal point of pathogenesis research in mice since it seems to be the important determinant of cell tropism, species specificity, host choice, cell tropism, and disease.

Virus replication is initiated with the Adding the stem protein into certain receptors within the host surface. To get MHV, the principal receptor was proven to function as carcinoembryonic antigen--cell adhesion molecule (CEACAM), also for its individual coronavirus, HCoV-229E, along with some other group 1 coronaviruses, the receptor is aminopeptidase N. The exact mechanics of entry and uncoating have to be described, but probably occur by fusion out of Vibroplex is via endocytic vesicles. To get wildtype MHV, entry and uncoating constitute a pH separate procedure that's most likely direct combination evidenced by means of a fusion peptide from the 1 protein. The comprehension of this area of the S1 part of coronavirus, which equates to receptors, has been the foundation for research resulting in the very current and quite quick identification of angiotensin-converting enzyme 2 (ACE 2) as a receptor to get SCoV.

The Upcoming different stage in the lifetime Cycle consists of also translation and proteolytic processing of viral replicase proteins in the entered genome RNA, followed by the creation of cytoplasmic replication complexes in conjunction with membranes. Replication complexes are considered to be sites of several phases of viral RNA transcription and replication, and maybe assembly of viral nucleocapsids. Viral assembly happens both independently and physically different from viral replication complexes at the endoplasmic-reticulum-Golgi-intermediate compartment (ERGIC), a transitional zone between overdue ER and Golgi. Even though the mechanics by which replication goods are sent to sites of the meeting remain to be ascertained, it's been proven that subpopulations of replicase proteins and the structural nucleocapsid (N) translocate in replication complexes into websites of gathering and might mediate the procedure in conjunction with mobile membrane/protein trafficking pathways (Bost et al., 2000). Virus meeting at the ERGIC entails interactions of genome RNA, N, and the tissue protein (M), and also the little tissue protein (E), leading to the budding of virions to the lumen of both ER/Golgi virosomes. Additional maturation of virus contamination occurs during motion throughout the Golgi, leading to virosomes full of older particles. Trafficking of this virosomes into the cell surface hasn't been well recognized but is supposed to happen through regular vesicle maturation and exocytic procedures. The result is that the nonlytic release of this huge majority of older virions to the extracellular space. For MHV

141

and many different coronaviruses that could immediately fuse with cells, then there's a feature and quickly detectable cytopathic effect of cell-cell mix into multinucleated syncytia. The generation of infectious virus lasts after nearly all cells have been fused. Syncytia were reported as a readout of both SCoV receptor expression and cell disease.

Viral Replication Complex Formation and Function

After entry and uncoating, the 5′ many replicase genes of this enter positive-strand RNA genome is translated into 2 co-amino terminal replicase polyproteins, which are co- along with post-translationally processed by viral proteinases to give 15 to 16 adult replicase proteins, along with intermediate precursors. The nascent replicase polyproteins and intermediate precursors likely mediate the creation of viral replication complexes at the host cell cytoplasm. Interestingly, the coronavirus replication demands constant replicase gene processing and processing during the life span to keep effective infection. Replication complexes of MHV are connected with double-membrane vesicles; also, most of the analyzed MHV replicase proteins are demonstrated to colocalize into replication complexes in the first time of discovery probably either by cartilage integration and from protein-protein along with protein-RNA interactions. Further, the replicase proteins probably mediate the procedure for double-membrane vesicle formation, probably by induction of cellular autophagy pathways (E. Prentice, unpublished results).

Coronavirus replication complexes Are websites for replicase gene translation and replicase polyprotein processing, and for viral RNA synthesis. Replicase receptor proteins probably contain positive-strand, negative-strand, subgenomic, and genomic RNA synthesis, in addition to procedures of capping, polyadenylation, RNA unwinding, template switching during viral RNA synthesis, along with the discontinuous transcription and transcription attenuation. The coronavirus replicase polyproteins and older replicase proteins represent the greatest and most varied repertoire of well-known and called different enzymatic purposes of almost any positive-strand RNA virus household. Until lately, of those 15 or even more adult replicase proteins, just the proteinase, RNA helicase, also RNA-dependent RNA polymerase actions were predicted or confirmed. With the introduction of SARS, broader bioinformatics investigations have led to forecasts of many additional functions included in RNA processing, such as methyltransferase and exonuclease activities. In spite of the addition of distant called connections, up to eight of these replicase proteins stay without called or supported purposes. In conclusion, it's very likely the coronaviruses have exploited their own innate capacity to synthesize proteins at the replicase gene using different roles in RNA processing and synthesis, in addition to proteins with particular roles in modification or induction in host cellular membrane biogenesis and trafficking, shipping of replication goods to websites of gathering, and potentially virus assembly. Therefore replicase translation, replicase polyprotein processing, and adult replicase proteins represent significant targets for disturbance using coronavirus replication, virus-cell interactions, or viral pathology.

Coronavirus Replicase Protein Expression and Performance

The proteinase actions for all Coronaviruses contain both papain-like proteinase (PLP) and also picornavirus 3C-like proteinase actions which are encoded inside the replicase polyproteins and mediate both cis and trans cleavage occasions. Due to the parallel growth of these proteinases, their cleavage sites, along with the hierarchical cleavage procedures, the proteolytic processing of this coronavirus replicase proteins might function as different regulatory and hereditary elements. Especially, you will find conserved and divergent areas of the replicase polyproteins with amino acid identity and similarity, together with the strings and called mature proteins, starting with all the 3C-like proteinases throughout the carboxy terminus of the replicase polyprotein keeping greater correlation and identity throughout the called proteins. By comparison, the amino-terminal third of this replicase shows the newest variation in proteins, including cleavage site places, and also the number of proteinases that mediate maturation processing. SCoV seems to get the overall association of, and also similar protein dimensions into, the group 2 coronaviruses like MHV inside this component of the genome. But, SCoV probably uses just 1 PLP to mediate the cleavages, like the category 3 coronavirus infectious bronchitis virus (IBV). Thus this area of the replicase can go through the maximum variability, indicating either the design of attachment functions that are flexible and conducive to adjustments or conversely class or host-specific functions that are susceptible to pressure to quickly shift.

Expression of Structural and Accessory Genes

Just the 5′ many replicase genes are Interpreted from the enter positive-strand genome RNA. The genome includes multiple different genes to the famous structural proteins , E, M, and N, in addition to some other genres such as proteins which were tagged as "non-structural" or "attachment" since they've been assumed not to be needed for replication, and aren't believed to be integrated into virions. MHV encodes half of those genes, whilst SCoV encodes potentially up to 11 attachment and structural genes, which are extracted from subgenomic mRNAs. Subgenomic RNA transcription occurs during minus-strand RNA synthesis by the purchase of those anti leader RNA sequences by the 5′ ending of the genome through homology into a

145

transcriptional regulatory sequence (TRS, also called an intergenic sequence), also necessitating a discontinuous action of this nascent minus-strand template along with polymerase complicated to obtain the chief. The results of transcription are that the creation of a "nested set" of all subgenomic negative-strand RNAs that contain the anti-leader sequences which function as templates for comparable dimension subgenomic mRNAs. This transcriptional strategy exhibits distinct genes since the 5' ORF in distinct mRNAs, all of which also include the 3' sequence downstream of this receptor, such as the 3' no translated region of the genome.

For MHV, genes , 5b, 6, and 7 Encode 1, E, M, and N, respectively. Period two, 4, and 5a aren't necessary for replication in society and are mutated to obstruct saying, deleted, or substituted with all noncoronavirus genes like GFP. Considering that all coronaviruses keep these enzymes in a variety of combinations in the surface of presumed stress for hereditary market and apparent deficiency of acts in RNA synthesis, so it's assumed that these genes function roles in alteration of host tissues, pathogenesis, or interactions with the immune system. SCoV encodes a bigger and more intricate collection of those genes than MHV or other coronaviruses, which might reflect its development in its initial creature host. Moreover, the record on a deletion within a few of the attachment genes in the human form of SCoV indicates that this might be a receptor involved in host adaptation or range for both replication and transmission in people.

Coronavirus Genetics

The genetics of coronavirus Replication and pathogenesis have mostly been analyzed using natural variations, Host range mutants, passaged virus, and mutagenized viruses chosen for Temperature sensitivity and particular phenotypes. Classical complementation of Works made it feasible to specify at least eight different groups such as MHV, With the majority of the complementation groups localized into the replicase gene. Taking Benefit of high levels of homologous RNA-RNA recombination and of course Host range determinants from the S protein, that the growth of targeted Recombination has enabled more defined and more thorough studies of this attachment And structural elements of MHV, transmissible gastroenteritis virus (TGEV), also Feline infectious peritonitis virus (FIPV). Studies with natural variations and Targeted recombination genetic research have shown that the protein is The significant determinant of host range, tropism, and pathogenesis; additional hereditary Components, maybe from the replicase, can influence these traits of Various coronaviruses. The ability of coronaviruses to alter server range, Transmission, pathogenesis, and disorder was shown in the lab Employing mobile virus and adaptation passing and continues to be shown in character by Natural versions of MHV, TGEV, and bovine coronavirus (BCOV), in addition to by Studies with heterologous viruses like canine coronavirus (CcoV) to Immunize cats from FIPV. Further, most targeted recombination research has Supported the genetic potency of this coronavirus genome and the capability of Coronaviruses to regain wild-type replication after deletions, mutations, Substitutions, and gene sequence rearrangements from the structural and attachment genes.

Challenges For genetic studies employing natural variations and mutants, especially in Defining the exact changes accountable for modified phenotypes, has restricted Advancement in clinical studies. Targeted recombination, though a robust method with Powerful choice, was restricted to studies of this 3′ 10 kb of this MHV Genome and can be restricted to the choice of viable recombinants. Lately, the Institution of "infectious clone" reverse genetic approaches for your coronaviruses TGEV (Transmissible Gastroenteritis Coronavirus), HCoV-229E, IBV, And MHV is now possible to examine the genetics of this whole Genome and each one the structural, attachment, and replicase genes. Approaches to "contagious cloning" have comprised full-blown cDNA clones of both TGEV genome in bacterial Artificial chromosomes, recombinant vaccinia viruses including full-blown cDNA clones of both HCoV-229E along with IBV genomes, and in vitro gathering plans for TGEV, MHV, and most lately, SCoV.

The in vitro assembly Strategy was Designed to overcome the battle of full-scale cDNA cloning of the TGEV and MHV genomes, which comprised "poisonous" areas in the replicase gene, leading to shaky or poisonous clones from E. coli. Subcloning of those areas required dividing the poisonous domains into different clones. The end result of this plan was that the cloning of the MHV genome to seven championships (A through G). To recover possible virus, the next approach is pursued: (1) cloned cDNA fragments have been derived from a plasmid with course 2 restriction enzymes which eliminate the comprehension site and render overhanging genomic arrangement; (two) excised fragments are ligated (constructed) in vitro; (3) transcription of full-length genomic RNA is pushed in vitro with a T7 promoter over the 5′ fragment A; (4) full-size genome RNA is electroporated into cells which are subsequently brushed onto a monolayer of naturally-occurring cells; also (5) cells have been monitored for cytopathic effect or carbohydrates, and also virus is retrieved from plaques or networking supernatant.

In vitro meeting has many Benefits For genetic research of this a big and complicated genome RNA. To begin with, genetic changes could be released and verified in stable tiny fragments with no demand to get a ~30kb genomic clone. Secondly, the cloned fragments ensure it is feasible to produce libraries of mutations that may quickly be analyzed in various combinations. Additional identification of putative second-site reversion mutations for right-handed introduced modifications could be introduced together with the initial mutation to verify their reversion possible. In conjunction with biochemical and cell imaging processes, additionally, it can research highly defective or deadly mutations from electroporated cells, so as to identify crucial determinants of replication. The in vitro assembly strategy was used to present marker mutations that are quiet for replication in society. Additionally, we've engineered mutations from the MHV replicase gene to specify the prerequisites for polyprotein processing and also to ascertain the use of particular replicase proteins at replication in society and also in pathogenesis in animals. Using this strategy, we've regained viruses with mutations in polyprotein cleavage sites and proteinase catalytic residues, and all of which have different phenotypes in protein processing, and viral growth, and viral RNA synthesis (unpublished results). Therefore, direct inverse genetic studies of this crucial replicase gene function could be achieved within the Vitro assembly of infectious clones.

Advances in SCoV Research

The rapid advancement in the Identification and characterization of SCoV since the etiologic agent of SARS was made possible from the simple fact that the virus grows well in society, also from the foundational study in coronaviruses that's been encouraged from the National Institutes of Health, the Multiple Sclerosis

Foundation, the U.S. Department of Agriculture, along with other organizations within the previous two decades. The use of knowledge regarding virus construction, genetics, hormone binding, virus entry, along with viral pathogenesis, is now feasible to aim the spike protein to the research of SCoV replication, pathogenesis, and immune reaction. The unusually fast identification of ACE 2 as a receptor for SARS has shown the foundational relevance of research of different coronaviruses. In the same way, comprehension of replicase gene expression, communicating, and called works have identified potential goals for structure/function research and potential therapeutic intervention. The research of coronavirus proteinase actions, cleavage website, and constructions were the foundation for studies resulting in the rapid conclusion of SCoV replicase polyprotein cleavage sites and 3CLpro crystal arrangement.

Application Of Reverse Genetics to Research of SCoV

Due to the possibility of Re-emergence of SARS, it's crucial to proceed with research in diagnostics, vaccines, and therapeutics such as SCoV. Experience with the development and application of reverse osmosis to research different coronaviruses led to the establishment of genetics for SCoV in weeks of the beginning of the international outbreak. How should the comprehension of different coronaviruses, the fast progress in the study with SCoV, and also the growth of reverse osmosis for SCoV be more

151

harnessed to attain these aims and assault these essential issues in SCoV replication, pathogenesis, and disease? Surely, using SCoV reverse osmosis, together with strong tissue culture methods and emerging animal models, generates the capacity to quickly answer questions regarding (1) determinants of virus growth in civilization (2) possible mechanics of transspecies adaptation; (3) sensitivity to escape from resistant and biochemical disturbance with replication; (4) determinants of virulence and pathogenesis; (5) mechanics of genome recombination and mutation; (6) acts of and prerequisites for replicase, structural, and attachment proteins; and (7) development of stably attenuated viruses to use as seed stocks such as an inactivated vaccine or examining because live-attenuated vaccines.

How then if these crucial Issues be researched while recognizing the capacity of SCoV to create acute illness, in addition to the prospect of rapid spread? To begin with, there's significant experience with different coronaviruses from attenuation of virus replication and pathogenesis, both with virus passing and from direct technology of modifications. Though coronavirus genome association, proteins, and replication seem more conducive to changes afterward previously believed, all fluctuations of chemical sequence, gene deletion, insertion, or mutagenesis thus far reported have contributed to viruses diminished in replication, pathogenesis or even both. Many of those attenuating modifications in MHV along with other coronaviruses are preserved in SCoV and so might be analyzed for probable attenuation from SCoV culture and animal models. Secondly, where there's apparent conservation of strings, themes, proteins, or putative works between SCoV and version viruses like MHV, brand new or untested modifications could be rapidly examined under BSL2 states in those form viruses, then immediately applied to SARS after their phenotypes are decided. Third, all use SCoV is going to be carried out just under BSL3 requirements. This would also apply to chimeric viruses, if or engineered by debut to the SCoV backdrop, or simply by introducing SCoV strings or proteins with predicted or known pathogenic effects into other coronavirus foundations. In the end, it's very important to build breeds of SCoV, which are attenuated and protected from reversion and recombination, to be utilized as the foundation for the research of additional replication and pathogenesis determinants and structure of virus chimeras. Such attenuated variations would offer extra defenses while allowing the use of strong genetic resources to the analysis of SCoV development, biology, illness, therapy, and prevention. In general, recently invigorated apps in other animal and human coronaviruses, together with the new study in SCoV, will shed significant new light with this virus household and possibly lead to greater comprehension of the possibility of a resurgence of SCoV or even the development of different coronaviruses into human inhabitants.

Prevention

There's currently no vaccine for Stop coronavirus disorder 2019 (COVID-19). The ideal approach to avoid illness is to prevent being vulnerable to the virus. However, since a reminder, CDC constantly urges regular preventative actions to help block the spread of respiratory ailments, such as:

Avoid close contact with those that are sick.

- Avoid touching your eyes, nose, and mouth area.
- Stay home when You're sick.
- Cover your cough or sneeze with a tissue, then throw the tissue from the garbage.
- Wipe and clean often touched surfaces and objects utilizing a normal family cleaning spray or wash.
- Practice CDC's recommendations for utilizing a facemask.
  - CDC doesn't recommend people that are well put on a facemask to protect themselves from respiratory ailments, such as COVID-19.
  - Facemasks ought to be employed by men and women who show indications of COVID-19 to help avoid the spread of this disease to other people. The usage of facemasks can also be critical for health employees and

individuals that are taking care of somebody in near configurations (at home or in a healthcare facility).

- Wash your hands frequently with soap and warm water for a minimum of 20 minutes, particularly after visiting the toilet; before ingestion; after blowing your nose, coughing, or sneezing.
  - If soap and water aren't easily available, utilize an alcohol-based hand sanitizer using 60% alcohol. Always wash hands with water and soap if hands are visibly dirty.

These are regular habits that can help stop the spread of many viruses. CDC will have special guidance for travellers.

Control and Prevention

Steps for protecting employees from Exposure to, and disease with, the book coronavirus, COVID-19 are contingent on the sort of task being done and vulnerability risk, such as possible for discussion with infectious individuals and pollution of the work environment. Employers must accommodate disease control plans based on comprehensive hazard evaluation, together with appropriate combinations of administrative and engineering controls, safe work procedures, and personal protective equipment (PPE) to reduce employee exposures. Several OSHA standards that are applicable to preventing occupational exposure to COVID-19 additionally need companies to train employees on components of disease prevention, such as PPE.

OSHA has developed this interim Advice to help avoid employee exposure to COVID-19.

U.S. Department of Defense

No matter particular exposure Dangers, adhering to excellent hand hygiene practices will help employees stay wholesome year-round.

General advice for all U.S. Employees and companies

For many employees, no matter Specific vulnerability risks, it's almost always a great practice to:

- Regularly wash your hands with water and soap for a minimum of 20 minutes. When soap and warm water are unavailable, make use of an impracticable hand wash at least 60% alcohol. Always wash hands, which are clearly fine.
- Avoid touching your eyes, nose, or mouth with unwashed hands.
- Avoid close contact with those that are sick.

The U.S. Centers for Disease Control And Prevention has generated interim advice for companies and companies to program for and react to COVID-19. The interim guidance is meant to help stop workplace accidents to severe respiratory disorders, such as COVID-19. The guidance also addresses concerns that can help companies prepare more prevalent, neighborhood outbreaks of COVID-19, in the event this type of transmission starts to happen. The advice is meant for non-healthcare configurations; health care employees and companies should consult advice specifically for them, under.

Interim advice for many U.S. Employees and employers of employees unlikely to possess occupational exposures to COVID-19

For many people on Earth, including most kinds of employees, the danger of disease with COVID-19 is presently low. This applies to U.S. employees not discussed elsewhere on this page (i.e., people not engaged in health care, deathcare, lab, airline, boundary security, or solid waste and wastewater management surgeries or global traveling to areas with continuing, person-to-person transmission of COVID-19). Such employees' exposure threat is very similar to that of their overall American people.

Employers and employees in surgeries Where there's not any particular vulnerability threat should stay conscious of the growing outbreak scenario. Changes in epidemic conditions may warrant extra precautions in certain offices not now highlighted within this advice.

Interim advice for U.S. employees and companies of employees with possible occupational exposures to COVID-19

Employees and companies involved in Health care, deathcare, lab, airline, boundary security, and solid waste and wastewater management surgeries, and global traveling to areas with continuing, person-to-person transmission of COVID-19 must stay conscious of the evolving outbreak scenario.

Employers should evaluate the dangers to that their employees could be exposed; assess the chance of vulnerability; and choose, employ, and make sure employees use controls to avoid exposure. Control measures might incorporate a blend of administrative and engineering controls, safe work practices, and PPE.

Discover and Isolate Suspected Cases

In most offices where vulnerability to That the COVID-19 may happen, prompt isolation and identification of potentially infectious people is an essential initial step in protecting employees, visitors, along with many others in the worksite.

- Instantly isolate individuals suspected of getting COVID-19. By way of instance, move possibly infectious folks to isolation chambers and shut the doors. In a plane, proceed possibly infectious folks to chairs away from crew and passengers, if you can and without compromising aviation security. In different worksites, proceed possibly infectious folks to a place away from employees, clients, and other people.

- Take action to restrict the spread of this individual's contagious respiratory secretions, such as by giving them a facemask and requesting them to use it, even if they could tolerate doing this. Notice: A surgical mask onto an individual or other ill person shouldn't be mistaken with PPE for an employee; the mask behaves to include potentially infectious respiratory secretions in origin (i.e., the individual's mouth and nose).

- If at all possible, isolate individuals suspected of getting COVID-19 separately from people with proven cases of this virus to stop additional transmissions, such as in screening, triage, or health care centers.

- Limit the number of employees entering isolation regions, for example, the area of a patient using suspected/confirmed COVID-19.

- Shield employees in close contact* with all the ill person by employing additional administrative and engineering management, safe work procedures, and PPE.

*CDC defines "near getting" as being roughly six (6) ft (about two (2) meters) in an infected individual or inside the area or maintenance region of an infected individual for an extended time whilst not sporting recommended PPE. Close contact also has cases where there is immediate contact with infectious secretions, although not sporting recommended PPE. Close contact normally does not consist of short term interactions, like walking past someone.

Flu Decontamination

Right Now, There's no proof The COVID-19 is dispersed through environmental conditions, like coming in contact with infected surfaces.

Since the transmissibility of COVID-19 from contaminated environmental surfaces and items isn't entirely understood, companies should carefully assess whether workplaces occupied by individuals suspected of getting virus might have been infected and whether they have to be decontaminated in reaction.

Outside of health and deathcare Facilities, there's typically no requirement to execute specific cleanup or decontamination of work surroundings if an individual suspected of getting the virus was present unless these surroundings are clearly contaminated with blood or other body fluids. In restricted cases where additional cleaning and decontamination could be required, consult U.S. Centers for Disease Control and Prevention (CDC) advice for cleansing and purification environments, such as those infected with another coronavirus.

Employees who run cleaning jobs Have to be protected from exposure to blood, specific human body fluids, and other potentially infectious substances covered by OSHA's Bloodborne Pathogens standard (29 CFR 1910.1030) and out of toxic substances used in those activities. In such scenarios, that the PPE (29 CFR 1910 Subpart I) and Hazard Communication (29 CFR 1910.1200) criteria may also use. Don't use pressurized air or water sprays to wash possibly contaminated surfaces, because these techniques can aerosolize infectious substance.

Watch the interim advice for Specific employee groups and their companies, under, for more info.

Employee Training

Train all employees with reasonably anticipated occupational exposure to COVID-19 (as explained within this document) regarding the sources of vulnerability to this virus, the dangers related to this exposure, and proper workplace protocols rather than block or lower the odds of vulnerability. Training should include advice about ways to isolate people who have suspected or verified COVID-19 or other infectious diseases, and also the way to report potential circumstances. Training has to be provided during scheduled workdays and free of charge to the worker.

Employees needed to use PPE needs to be trained. This practice involves when to utilize PPE; exactly what PPE is required, how to correctly don (put on), utilize, and also doff (remove) PPE; the way to correctly eliminate disinfect, inspect for damage, and keep PPE; and also the constraints of PPE. Applicable standards incorporate the PPE (29 CFR 1910.132), Eye and Face Protection (29 CFR 1910.133), Employed Security (29 CFR 1910.138), and Occupational Safety (29 CFR 1910.134) criteria. The OSHA site delivers a number of training videos on respiratory defense.

If the possibility exists for Vulnerability to individual bloodstream, specific human body fluids, or other potentially infectious substances , employees should receive the training needed by the Bloodborne Pathogens (BBP) standard (29 CFR 1910.1030), such as advice about how to identify tasks which may involve exposure as well as the processes, including engineering controls and work practices, and PPE, to decrease exposure. Additional Details about OSHA's BBP training policies and regulations can be obtained for companies and employees on the

OSHA Bloodborne Pathogens and Needlestick Prevention Safety and Health Topics page.

OSHA's Coaching and Reference Materials Library includes reference and training materials created from the OSHA Directorate of Training and Instruction in addition to links to other associated websites. The substances recorded for Bloodborne Pathogens, PPE, Respiratory Protection, and SARS can offer extra material for companies to utilize in preparing training for their employees.

OSHA's Personal Protective Gear Security and Health Topics page also offers advice on instruction in the use of PPE.

Interim guidance for specific employee Their companies

This section Offers information For specific employee groups and their companies who might have possible flaws to COVID-19. Guidance for every employee group normally follows the selection of controllers, such as engineering controls and administrative controls, safe work practices, and PPE. But not all sorts of controllers are supplied in each part; in these scenarios, employers and employees should consult with the interim general advice for U.S. employees and employers of employees with possible occupational exposures to COVID-19, over.

Treatment

There's no specific antiviral Treatment advocated for COVID-19. Individuals with COVID-19 must receive supportive services to help alleviate symptoms. For severe cases, therapy must incorporate care to encourage critical organ functions.

Individuals that think they Might Have been Vulnerable to COVID-19 must call their healthcare provider promptly.

Coronavirus disorder (COVID-19) information for the General Public

Fundamental protective measures from the brand-new coronavirus

Remain alert to the Most Recent information About the COVID-19 outbreak, on the WHO site, and throughout your federal and local public health jurisdiction. COVID-19 remains impacting mostly individuals in China with a few outbreaks in different nations. Many individuals who get infected experience moderate disease and recuperate, but it may be severe for many others. Look after Your Wellbeing and protect the others by performing the following:

Wash your hands regularly

Often and thoroughly wash your Palms using an alcohol-based hand wash or scrub them with water and soap.

Why? Scrub your hands with soap and warm water, or utilizing alcohol-based hand moisturize kills germs, which could be in your palms.

Maintain social networking

Keep at least 1 meter (3 ft) Distance between yourself and anybody who's coughing or coughing.

Why? Whenever someone coughs or sneezes, they squirt little liquid droplets in their mouth or nose, which might contain the virus. If you're too near, you are able to breathe at the droplets, for example, the COVID-19 virus in the event the individual coughing gets the disorder.

Avoid touching eyes, mouth and nose

Why? Hands Signature several surfaces and may pick up viruses. Once contaminated, palms can move the virus into your eyes, mouth, or nose. From that point, the virus may put in your entire body and can cause you to be sick.

Exercise respiratory hygiene

Be sure to personally, as well as the folks around You, follow good respiratory hygiene. This usually means covering your nose and mouth with your flexed knee or tissue whenever you sneeze or cough. Then eliminate the tissue that is used instantly.

Why? Droplets spread contamination. By carrying out good respiratory hygiene that you shield the folks around you from germs like influenza, cold and COVID-19.

When you have fever, cough and difficulty breathing, seek medical attention early

Stay home if you're feeling unwell. Should you Have a fever, cough and difficulty breathing, seek medical care, and telephone ahead of time. Follow the instructions of the regional health authority.

Why? National and local governments may have the most current info on the specific situation in your town. Calling beforehand will permit your healthcare provider to rapidly direct you into the ideal wellness facility. This can even protect you and assist in preventing the spread of germs and other illnesses.

Stay educated and follow information Supplied by your physician

Stay informed on the most recent Changes about COVID-19. Follow the information provided by your own physician, your local and national public health jurisdiction, or your company about the best way best to guard yourself and others out of COVID-19.

Why? National and local governments may have the most current advice on if COVID-19 is dispersing in your town. They are best positioned to advise about what folks in your town ought to be doing to protect themselves.

Security measures for men who Are in or have recently seen (past 14 days) places where COVID-19 is dispersing

- Practice the advice outlined above.

- Stay at home when you start to feel nostalgic, despite moderate symptoms like headache and minor runny nose before you recuperate. Why? Preventing contact with other people and visits to health centers will make it possible for these centers to function more efficiently and also help safeguard you and other people from potential COVID-19 and other germs.

- Should you develop fever, fever, and difficulty breathing, seek medical advice immediately as this might be due to respiratory disease or other serious illness. Telephone beforehand and inform your supplier of any travel or contact with travellers. Why? Calling beforehand will permit your well-being care provider to rapidly direct you into the ideal wellness facility. This may also help prevent the potential spread of COVID-19 along with other germs.

CONCLUSION

A brand new and deadly virus has reared Its horrible head, causing grave concern among the worldwide health community. HCov-EMC, aka Human Coronavirus - Erasmus Medical Center, has been 1st known in mid-afternoon 2012. This deadly strain of coronavirus is seemingly highly deadly - so much 5 of those 11 understand victims of the fatal disease have expired. This virus is somewhat like a strain of coronavirus seen in bat populations. Unfortunately, it seems that this new and lethal virus has made the jump from animals to people, and much more upsetting, lately a human to human transmission has occurred.

The very first recorded victim was Identified in June 012 if a 60-year-old male appeared at a Jidda Saudi Arabia clinic with influenza-like symptoms and trouble breathing. In a couple of days of entry into the hospital, that this individual died of kidney failure and acute pneumonia. In the previous seven months, 11 more instances are identified, such as one in England in ancient 2013. This specific instance of HCov-EMC was especially disturbing to global infectious disease investigators and WHO (World Health Organization) since the British sufferer apparently contracted the deadly and new coronavirus from his dad, who had recently travelled to the Middle East. The virus's clear ability to jump from animal to person then immediately from human to human is quite disturbing.

The Indications of HCov-EMC disease Are influenza-like, such as fever, and cough, and difficulty breathing, and which rapidly evolves to acute pneumonia and renal (kidney) failure. Public health has seemed a warning to the global community advising all healthcare centers and doctors to know about and to record any abnormal respiratory ailments. This new coronavirus is comparable to SARS (severe acute respiratory disease) and maybe even more deadly and more contagious. While the very low rate of the disease so far suggests that HCov-EMC now has a minimal transmission speed - caregivers are extremely worried at any given time this deadly new breed of coronavirus may mutate into an extremely infectious disease that may quickly spread person-to-person worldwide.

Only time will tell if That the HCov-EMC will or won't be our next jolt and if we have developed the ideal antibiotics to prevent it. The gain in the speed of disease transmission from animal to people has been alert the global wellness community. With the rise in global travel, we still continue to find a rise in the mutation and spread of person into animal diseases(zoonoses) that arise in distant regions of the planet (where near human/animal contact happens more often). At any time, one of that brand new and lethal disease could cause a fatal global plague. It's very important that we're awake and ready to face that which seems to be inescapable.

After clusters of infection instances of No known reason were epidemiologically linked into your fish and 'moist' monster wholesale food market at Wuhan, China, three teams worked tirelessly to recognize the offender. To begin with, researchers in Shanghai, Wuhan, Beijing, and Sydney utilized metagenomic RNA sequencing to recognize the unknown coronavirus at a sample by one individual who had worked in the marketplace. This group pitched a draft genome sequence from the publicly accessible GenBank chain repository 10 January, so the present variant was sprinkled on 17 January.

Around Precisely the Same time, a Rapid-response team dispatched by the Australian Center for Disease Control and Prevention reported they had been isolated and cultivated that a novel coronavirus by bronchoalveolar lavage fluid of three individuals also recognized it as the likely origin of the epidemic. Electron microscopy observations found a normal coronavirus morphology; light microscopy operate revealed it'd cytopathic effects on human airway epithelial cells. Genome sequencing demonstrated the virus shared above 85% sequence identity with a famous SARS-like coronavirus found in bats. On 12 January, this team deposited three additional genome sequences at the open entry database International Initiative on Sharing All of Influenza Data (GISAID).

The third set of scientists located At Wuhan and Beijing, characterized and identified the exact same virus at a further five patients with acute pneumonia and hauled five more genomes with GISAID. They also revealed that the virus employs angiotensin-converting receptor II (ACE2) to get entrance to host cells, as did SARS-CoV, the breed that resulted in 2002--2003 epidemic, which infected 8,096 individuals and caused 774 deaths.

Several global groups have Been operating from those string information to design primers for polymerase chain reaction (PCR) tests to encourage international public health labs at the Lack of a commercial evaluation for SARS-CoV-2 (previously 2019-nCoV). The laboratory of Christian Drosten, in the Institute of Virology, Charité University Hospital, Berlin, Together with academic collaborators from Europe and Hong Kong, printed Particulars of a real-time PCR (RT-PCR) analytical evaluation and workflow to 23 January, Which finds SARS-CoV-2 and distinguishes it in SARS-CoV. The group confirmed the evaluation in the lack of SARS-CoV-2 isolates or individual samples but affirmed Its specificity from 297 clinical trials in patients with different other Respiratory ailments. This formed the foundation of imports of 250,000 kits That the World Health

Organization (WHO) discharged to 159 labs across the world in recent weeks.

Meanwhile, A team at Hong Kong University have grown 2 one-step quantitative RT Reverse transcription PCR tests targeting the open reading frame 1b (ORF1b) along with also the southern regions of the viral genome based on the initial sequence Deposited at GenBank; those two evaluations have been confirmed with two clinical Specimens obtained from individuals infected by SARS-CoV-2. The evaluations are Specifically made to spot numerous viruses from the arbovirus subgenus. To that, SARS-CoV-2 belongs, provided a shortage of information on the ideology of SARS-CoV-2 in people as well as animals. As no additional sarbecoviruses are proven to be Circulating in humans, a positive evaluation could be regarded as an affirmation that an Issue is infected with either SARS-CoV-2 or even a connected animal virus. The N receptor assay Is advocated as a screening test, and also the ORF1b evaluation is advocated as a confirmatory test. The diagnostic algorithm is comparable to that followed for its Middle East respiratory syndrome (MERS) coronavirus, which was diagnosed In Saudi Arabia in 2012. "

As opposed to develop bespoke PCR evaluations, IDbyDNA is just one of a couple of organizations using metagenomic lipoic acid analysis as a routine diagnostic and surveillance instrument. Its present Explify Respiratory evaluation, which can be a laboratory-developed (or even 'homebrew') evaluation, may identify over 900 cancerous tumors, such as viruses, bacteria, viruses, fungi and parasites, and by assessing impartial metagenomic data acquired from individual samples using a massive repository of sequence information. It could already discover SARS-CoV-2 pressure. "We've updated our information together with the brand-new coronavirus and have been in the process of revalidating," The alterations are on the data analysis aspect " This is, he states, a simpler procedure than upgrading an actual assay. The true data evaluation takes under an hour the turnaround time from receipt of sample to check outcome is 36 hours. Although more costly compared to PCR testing, the decreasing prices of sequencing can help democratize this strategy. The business is promoting technologies in addition to its testing solutions.

Assessing the outbreak by assessing the phylogenetic relationships between distinct SARS-CoV-2 genomes. RNA viruses possess an error-prone replication procedure, along with the genetic variants which are introduced comprise a molecular clock that may provide insights to the first emergence and continuing development of the virus. "The circadian clock provides a method of altering the genetic changes to period," he states. A first analysis, dependent on 90 publicly available genomes, indicates that SARS-CoV-2 appeared long until the very first instances of disease in Wuhan happened. "It does not predate the time of the illness detection that far.

Epidemiologists also have accommodated digital surveillance programs to monitor the new coronavirus epidemic by automatically tracking unstructured and structured digital data in the official and unofficial resources. The middle for Systems Science and Engineering at Johns Hopkins University has generated an on-line dashboard to picture and monitor reported instances of SARS-CoV-2 in actual time. The underlying data will be publicly available to scientists via a GitHub repository. The dash's main supply is DXY, an internet source conducted by members of the Chinese health care community, that aggregate media and official reports about the creation of the outbreak. HealthMap.org, developed over a decade back to monitor infectious disease outbreaks and has released an interface special for SARS-CoV-2. Crowdsourcing and automatic data retrieval also have been exploited to create a shared digital line-up for monitoring the SARS-CoV-2 outbreak, case by case. On 19 February, the record comprised demographic, geographical, and clinical details about over 7,800 different scenarios, which permits investigators to run analyses to comprehend patterns of spread. "Lots of classes are utilizing the information, so that is one reassuring thing," says Moritz Krämer, research fellow in Department of Zoology, Oxford University, that put up the source.

Myriad uncertainties still surround the trajectory of this outbreak. On the flip side, containment attempts beyond China seem, so much, to become prosperous. The amount of verified cases in different states remains low, and there's not much evidence for this stage of widespread network transmission. Back in China, however, and especially at Hubei province -- that the epicenter of the epidemic, which stays in lockdown -- that the film remains unclear. Nearly all cases still haven't solved. In addition, the magnitude of the 'iceberg' is undefined: it's still too early to learn whether additional unnoticed reservoirs of disease stay.